Vascular Biology in Clinical Practice

Vascular Biology in Clinical Practice

- ◆ **Hypertension**
- ◆ **Hyperlipidemia**
- ◆ **Atherosclerosis**
- ◆ **Coronary Heart Disease**

Mark C. Houston, MD, FACP
Clinical Professor of Medicine
Vanderbilt University School of Medicine

American Society of Hypertension (ASH)
Specialist in Clinical Hypertension

Director, Hypertension Institute
Saint Thomas Medical Group
Saint Thomas Hospital and Health Services
Nashville, Tennessee

Forewords by Carlos M. Ferrario, MD, FACA, FACC
and Jonathan Ravid Jaffe, MD, FACC, FAHA

HANLEY & BELFUS, INC. / Philadelphia

Publisher: HANLEY & BELFUS, INC.
               Medical Publishers
               210 South 13th Street
               Philadelphia, PA 19107
               (215) 546-7293; 800-962-1892
               FAX (215) 790-9330
               Website: http://www.hanleyandbelfus.com

To order additional copies of this book or to obtain information about the purchase of a
large quantity, please contact the publisher at the numbers listed above.

Library of Congress Cataloging-in-Publication Data

Houston, Mark C.
     Vascular biology in clinical practice/written by Mark C. Houston.
     p. ; cm.
     Includes index.
     ISBN 1-56053-488-5
     1. Blood-vessels—Diseases—Handbooks, manuals, etc. I. Title.
     [DNLM: 1. Vascular Diseases—Handbooks. 2. Blood
     Vessels—physiology—Handbooks. 3. Blood Vessels—physiopathology—Handbooks. WG
     39 H843v 2001]
     RC691 .H68 2002
     616.1'3—dc21   2001026405

Vascular Biology in Clinical Practice

                                                   ISBN 1-56053-488-5

Last digit is the print number: 9 8 7 6 5 4 3 2

Contents

Acknowledgments

Special thanks to the following individuals:

For review of and comments on the Handbook
> Dr. Carlos Ferrario
> Dr. Jonathan Jaffe
> Dr. Jordan Asher
> Dr. Ralph Hawkins

For administrative and secretarial support
> Sherry Gill

For all my medical staff
> Laurie, Sandra, Mary, Linda, Roanna, Sharon, Robin, Jill and Monica

For the gracious forewords:
> Carlos M. Ferrario, MD, FACA, FACC
> Dewitt-Cordell Professor of Surgical Sciences
> Professor of Physiology and Pharmacology
> Director, The Hypertension and Vascular Disease Center
> Wake Forest University School of Medicine
> Winston-Salem, North Carolina
> President and CEO
> The Consortium for Southeastern Hypertension Control

> Jonathan Ravid Jaffe, MD, FACC, FAHA
> Director, The Lipid and Hypertension Center of Excellence
> Fort Lauderdale, Florida
> Vice-President, Florida Lipid Associates
> Orlando, Florida
> American Society of Hypertension (ASH)
> Specialist in Clinical Hypertension

Preface

An understanding of vascular biology has become crucial for the practicing clinician to optimally treat patients with vascular disease as well as to prevent vascular problems and target organ damage. Recent research has clearly demonstrated that hypertension, hyperlipidemia, diabetes mellitus, coronary heart disease, congestive heart failure, cerebrovascular accidents, renal disease, and generalized atherosclerosis are intimately tied to endothelial dysfunction and vascular smooth muscle dysfunction. An appreciation of traditional, emerging, and nontraditional cardiovascular risk factors and how they impact vascular biology has opened new insights into pathophysiology, clinical outcomes, prevention, and treatment with both nonpharmacologic and pharmacologic approaches.

These common diseases should be viewed as primarily a disease of the blood vessel. Therapy should be directed toward the primary disease, but even more importantly, it should be directed toward improving blood vessel health–both structure and function. Although many drugs are effective in improving a primary endpoint such as blood pressure, lipids or glucose, their effects on vascular structure and function vary dramatically. The means by which treatment occurs in hypertension, hyperlipidemia, diabetes mellitus, coronary heart disease, congestive heart failure, or other cardiovascular disease is as important or more important than reaching a surrogate goal for that particular disease.

The purpose of this book is to provide clinicians, researchers, medical interns, residents, students, and other interested health care professionals with an up-to-date, easy to understand, readily accessible vascular biology handbook that spans the gamut of current basic, clinical, and treatment aspects. It is my hope that the concise summaries, tables, diagrams and brief text will provide a stimulating and valuable learning experience that will make it intellectually gratifying and fun to treat patients with cardiovascular disease. Ultimately, our goal is to help our patients, and I believe this handbook will help you to treat them to the best of your ability.

Mark C. Houston, M.D., F.A.C.P.
Associate Clinical Professor of Medicine
Vanderbilt University Medical School
Director, Hypertension Institute and Vascular Biology
Saint Thomas Medical Group
Saint Thomas Hospital and Health Services
Nashville, Tennessee

American Society of Hypertension (ASH)
Specialist in Clinical Hypertension

Consortium for Southeastern Hypertension Control
(COSEHC) designated Cardiovascular Center of
Excellence

Foreword I

Atherosclerosis, the leading cause of death in Western societies and emerging economies, has remained at the forefront of the efforts to improve the longevity of human life and reduce the ever-escalating costs of health care. Molecular biology, the introduction of gene technology, and genomic research have had an incredible impact on advancing knowledge of the processes that account for the evolution of the disease. The vascular endothelium has been identified as the fundamental cornerstone of a new understanding of the disease's mechanisms and, perhaps, is the earliest target for the initiation of the disease process. With this knowledge, it has become increasingly apparent that the dysfunction of the vascular endothelium and the mechanisms that support these events constitute a generalized disturbance of the endocrine function that this component of the vascular system plays in the regulation of vascular tone and perfusion pressure. The clinical benefits gained by this knowledge have translated into the introduction of new pharmacologic therapeutic modalities targeting angiotensin II, endothelin 1, and the rate of lipid peroxidation, advances in interventional cardiology, and the engineering of techniques for the local delivery of genes to sites of vascular disease.

This book has succeeded in synthesizing the rapid and ever-changing knowledge base in this budding field of vascular medicine. The well-organized chapters and the succinct but complete documentation of the data ensure the excellence of this book and guarantee its value for the practicing physician. The text has managed to preserve a proper balance between basic science and clinical medicine. Dr. Houston's efforts to amalgamate the process of atherogenesis as a reflection of a "mosaic" of mechanisms that affect vascular health reflect a cutting-edge approach to the problem and should be of immense value in helping clinicians to appropriately manage patients at risk for cardiovascular events.

While the pace of progress in cardiology is breathtaking, this book is unlikely to become obsolete. In weaving the biologic events associated with cardiovascular outcomes as components of a disease process for which high blood pressure, dyslipidemia, and insulin resistance reflect the expression of a fundamental underlying neurohormonal defect at the vascular wall, the author has articulated a case for a global management of cardiovascular ailments and ensured that the arguments presented will pass the test of time. Owing to the book's single authorship, the unifying theme of vascular dysfunction remains focused and clear throughout the 17 chapters that the book contains. This is an exemplary book that will serve well all professionals caring for cardiac patients and be a valuable reference source for those who wish to broaden their knowledge of cardiovascular medicine.

Carlos M. Ferrario, MD, FACA, FACC
Professor and Director
The Hypertension and Vascular Disease Center
Wake Forest University School of Medicine
Winston-Salem, North Carolina

President and CEO
The Consortium for Southeastern Hypertension Control

Foreword II

Rapid development of new technologies has become a given in modern medicine. Nowhere is this more important than in vascular biology. The vast majority of people in our industrialized, urbanized society will either become ill or die from occlusive vascular disease. The number one cause of death in both men and women in the western world overwhelmingly is coronary artery disease. The leading and most expensive cause of disability is cerebrovascular disease. Our understanding of the basic biology and subsequently of the pathobiology of vascular tissue has been revolutionized by the newer concepts of endothelial cell biology. The past 20 years has witnessed the growth of endothelium as a single organ despite its vast surface area.

Understanding normal endothelial physiology and then the environmental triggering of endothelial dysfunction has become essential to the early detection of vascular disease as well as to appropriate and aggressive risk modification in established vascular disease. Nowhere have basic concepts and philosophical constructs changed as fast as in this evolving field. With each passing year, the mechanisms for triggers such as hypertension, dyslipidemia, diabetes mellitus, cigarette smoking, and physical inactivity, as well as the newer identifiable triggers such as homocysteine, lipoprotein (a), oxidative stress, and even infectious agents, have become better understood. Better understanding of these mechanisms allows new targets for therapeutic intervention and manipulation.

In this text, Dr. Mark Houston has created a new source of vitally important cutting-edge information for healthcare providers. Dr. Houston is the Director of the Hypertension Institute, Saint Thomas Hospital, Nashville, Tennessee. Not only is he a practicing physician, a national and international authority in hypertension and endothelial vascular biology, but he is also actively involved in research of all aspects of these entities. In this exciting and well-written book, detailed descriptions of endothelial function and dysfunction, as well as the current understanding of the renin-angiotensin system and its role in hypertension, atherosclerosis, cardiovascular disease and oxidative stress, are elucidated. This book is definitively the most current and up-to-date review available. Dr Houston takes a subject that until recently has been esoteric and research oriented, and makes it understandable and clinically relevant for the practicing physician and healthcare giver.

Jonathan Ravid Jaffe, MD, FACC, FAHA
Director, The Lipid and Hypertension Center of Excellence
Fort Lauderdale. Florida
Vice-President, Florida Lipid Associates
Orlando, Florida

American Society of Hypertension (ASH)
Specialist in Clinical Hypertension

Dedication

To my dedicated and loving parents, Rupert R. Houston and Mary Ruth Houston, who made it possible for me to achieve my goals and dreams.

To my beloved wife, Laurie, who loves and understands me for who I am, and who steadfastly supports me.

To my wonderful children, Helen, Bo, John and Kelly, who make me proud and whom I love dearly.

To my God who blessed me in all things.

Chapter 1
Spectrum of Cardiovascular Disease

Cardiovascular Disease in Western Countries and Worldwide[6]

Cardiovascular disease (CVD) accounts for the majority of morbidity and mortality in western countries and in the world.

➤ CVD accounts for 30% of deaths worldwide:

➤ CHD: No. 1 cause of death
CVA: No. 4 cause of death

CVD is Predominantly an Atherosclerotic Vascular Disease

Atherosclerosis begins at an early age[42,43,45]

➤ Pathobiological Determinants of Atherosclerosis in Youth (PDAY) study (ages 15–19 at autopsy)[42]
60% with cholesterol deposits in abdominal aorta
60% with fatty streaks in right coronary artery

➤ Korean War Soldiers at Autopsy[43]
Advanced CHD found at average age of 22

➤ Holman study[45]
Fatty streaks in aorta: 1st decade
Fatty streaks in coronary arteries: 2nd decade
Fibrous plaques/CHD: 2nd–3rd decade

Key Concepts in Endothelial Dysfunction, Atherosclerosis, Cardiovascular Disease, and CHD

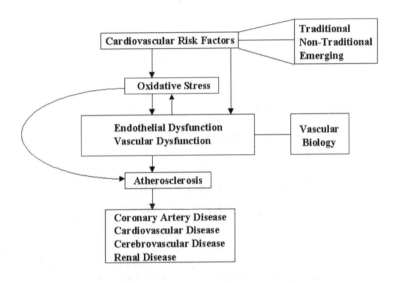

Oxidative stress to the blood vessel plays a major role in directly inducing endothelial dysfunction, vascular smooth muscle dysfunction, and atherosclerosis. Thus, oxidative stress is the mediator between cardiovascular risk factors and target organ damage.

The Hypertension Syndrome—It's More than Just Blood Pressure[111,112,113]

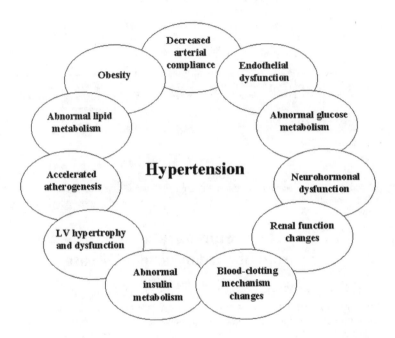

It is estimated that over 70% of patients with genetic hypertension have one or more of the coexisting metabolic or functional disorders that increase the risk of vascular damage, atherosclerosis, and target organ damage.

New Treatment Approach

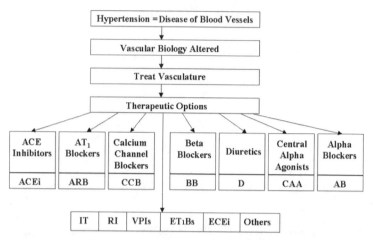

IRA, Imidazolidine receptor antagonist; RI, renin inhibitor; VPI, vasopeptidase inhibitor; ET1B, endothelin receptor blocker type B; ECEI, endothelin-converting enzyme inhibitor.

Summary
Spectrum of Cardiovascular Disease

Atherosclerosis starts at an early age in the US. CHD remains the number one cause of death in western countries. Traditional and new risk factors for CHD influence oxidative stress in the vascular system, which alters vascular biology and leads to endothelial dysfunction and vascular smooth muscle dysfunction. Clinical sequelae such as CHD, CVA, CHF, and renal insufficiency are increased as a result of this dysfunction.

Hypertension is one of the major risk factors for cardiovascular and cerebrovascular disease. Hypertension is a syndrome characterized by numerous metabolic and structural abnormalities in over 70% of patients. These abnormalities contribute to the high incidence of cardiovascular disease in hypertensive patients.

Treatment of hypertension with both nonpharmacologic and pharmacologic therapy must be directed at the blood vessels to improve vascular health. Since vascular biology is altered, an understanding of the pathology and pathogenesis of vascular and endothelial dysfunction is paramount in order to select the most appropriate treatment to prevent and reduce target organ damage that is a consequence of hypertension, hyperlipidema, diabetes mellitus, and other diseases.

Chapter 2
Historical Aspects of Atherosclerosis and Vascular Biology

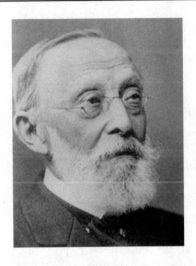

Rudolph Ludwig Carl Virchow (1821–1902)

(Photo from Simmons J: Rudolph Virchow and the cell doctrine. In The Scientific 100—A Ranking of the Most Influential Scientists, Past and Present. New Jersey, Carol Publishing Group, 1996.)

The renowned German physician and pathologist was the first to recognize and describe the pathogenesis of atherosclerosis as an inflammatory disease of the endothelium in 1845.

➢ Atherosclerosis pathogenesis (**endarteritis deformans**): Atheroma is a product of an inflammatory process within the intima (1845)

➢ Atherosclerosis is a reaction to injury and inflammation within the arterial wall

➢ **Cell doctrine** (1850)

Historical:
Endothelium and Nitric Oxide

➤ **Furchgott and Zawadzki** discovered the obligatory role played by endothelial cells in the relaxation of isolated arteries (vascular smooth muscle cells) of the rabbit in response to exogenous acetylcholine in 1980. They proposed endothelium-derived relaxing factor (EDRF) and received the Nobel Prize for Medicine and Physiology in 1998. (Furchgott RF, Zawadzki JV: The obligatory role of endothelial cells in the relaxation of arterial smooth muscle by acetylcholine. Nature 1980; 288:373–376.)

➤ **Palmer et al.** identified EDRF as nitric oxide (NO) in 1987. (Palmer RM, Ferrige AG, Moncada S: Nitric oxide release accounts for the biological activity of endothelium-derived relaxing factor. Nature 1987; 327:524–526.)

Summary
Historical Aspects

Recent clinical and basic scientific research has confirmed what Virchow described in 1845: that atherosclerosis is an inflammatory disease of the arterial wall and a reaction to injury from numerous inciting events. "Endarteritis deformans" described well our present view of endothelial dysfunction and vascular smooth muscle dysfunction.

Chapter 3
The Blood Vessel Structure

The Arterial Wall

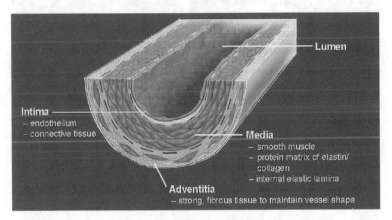

(Modified from Ross R: Atherosclerosis—an inflammatory disease. N Engl J Med 1999; 340:115–126, and Mulvany MJ, Aalkjaer C: Structure and function of small arteries. Physiol Rev 1990; 70:921–961.)

The walls of the artery consist of the intima, media, and adventitia.

The **intima**, the smooth inner lining of the vessel, comprises the endothelium and underlying connective tissue. Metabolically active endothelial cells line the lumen.

The middle layer, the **media or muscularis**, comprises smooth muscle cells (SMCs) that are surrounded by an extracellular protein matrix containing collagen, elastin fibers, fibroblasts, and an internal elastic lamina. Small arteries contain greater proportions of smooth muscle than large arteries. The media of large arteries (e.g., the aorta) has a relatively large amount of elastic tissue.

The **adventitia**, or outer layer of the arterial wall, comprises connective tissue that acts to maintain the shape of the vessel and limit distention.

The structural heterogeneity in large vs. intermediate vs. small vessels is potentially important in terms of disease processes and therapeutic responsiveness.

Endothelium[1,3,4]

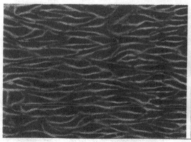 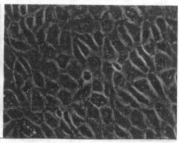

Physiologic Arterial
Hemodynamic Shear Stress
($^{\tau}$s>15 dyne/cm^2)

Low Arterial
Hemodynamic Shear Stress
($^{\tau}$s~ ± 0-4 dyne/cm^2)

The **vascular endothelium** under normal, healthy physiologic conditions forms a contiguous sheet of organized monolayer polyhedral cells that become disorganized at extremes of hemodynamic shear stress (hypotension and hypertension).

Endothelial cells create a conduit that separates blood from and allows blood to flow through tissues. Small vessels, capillaries, are primarily made of endothelial cells, while larger vessels have additional components, including connective tissue and smooth muscle, that add strength and tone to the vessel.

The endothelium is a living organ with multiple functions in addition to forming a barrier between the blood and the tissues. The endothelial cells are tightly interlocked so that passage of products from the blood occurs through the endothelial cell. The endothelial cells are both a passive filter and a metabolically active organ that secretes substances into and out of the blood and the underlying vascular smooth muscle to regulate the local milieu.

Vascular Endothelium

Size[1]

- Largest endocrine organ
- Largest organ in the body
- Over 14,000 ft^2 surface area
- $6\frac{1}{2}$ tennis courts in surface area
- 5 x heart size in mass
- Weight is 2 kg
- Metabolically active
- Role of tight and gap junctions
- Selective, passive permeability

Definition[1,3,4,6,55,67,105]

- Continuous sheet of parallel, polyhedral cells (3–4 μm thick)
- Monolayer interface between blood vessel and blood
- Releases vasoactive substances that regulate endothelial function, vascular smooth muscle (VSM), and circulating blood cells
- Endocrine, autocrine, paracrine, and intracrine functions
- Major function: Maintain appropriate **vasomotor tone**, especially in coronary arteries and systemic resistance arteries (i.e., homeostatic balance)

Summary
Blood Vessel Structure

The human blood vessel is composed of the *lumen* (blood elements), the *intima* (endothelium and connective tissue), the *media* (vascular smooth muscle, elastin, collagen), and the *adventitia* (fibrous tissue). The endothelium is thus the largest organ and the largest endocrine organ in the body. Its strategic location, its metabolic activity, and its endocrine, paracrine, autocrine, and intracrine functions explain the ability of the endothelial cells to affect blood constituents and vascular smooth muscle cell function and structure.

Chapter 4
Endothelial Function[1,4,9]

- Primary function: **Maintain vascular homeostasis**
- "Endothelial Function" = Endothelium-dependent vasodilation (EDV)
- Balance of opposing forces and functions
- Bidirectional effects with vasoactive secretions

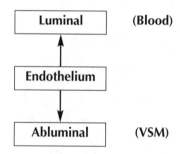

Vascular Endothelium: A Multifunctional Interface

Vital Functions of Vascular Endothelium:[105]

- Blood-compatible container
- Selective permeability barrier
- Monitor and transducer of blood-borne signals
- Source and target of biologic response modifiers
- Integrator of local pathophysiologic milieu
- Dynamic regulation of:
    - Hemostasis and thrombosis
    - Vascular tone
    - Vascular growth and remodeling
    - Inflammatory and immune reactions

Vascular Endothelium: Strategic Anatomic Position[6,105]

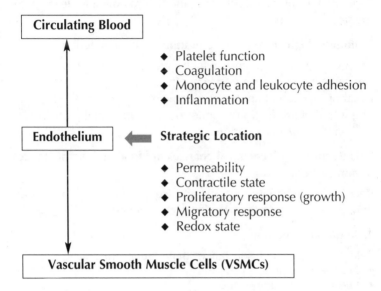

Circulating Blood

- ◆ Platelet function
- ◆ Coagulation
- ◆ Monocyte and leukocyte adhesion
- ◆ Inflammation

Endothelium ⟸ **Strategic Location**

- ◆ Permeability
- ◆ Contractile state
- ◆ Proliferatory response (growth)
- ◆ Migratory response
- ◆ Redox state

Vascular Smooth Muscle Cells (VSMCs)

The endothelium mantains vascular health and homeostatic balance.

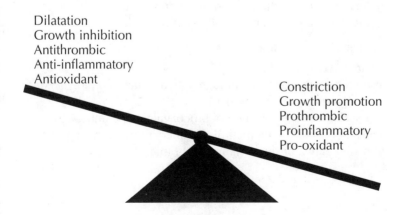

Dilatation
Growth inhibition
Antithrombic
Anti-inflammatory
Antioxidant

Constriction
Growth promotion
Prothrombic
Proinflammatory
Pro-oxidant

Functions of the Vascular Endothelium[4]

1. Highly selective permeable barrier

Regulation of plasma fluid, ions, and macromolecules from and to the vascular space

2. Immunologic, enzymatic, and inflammatory function

Production of interleukin-1, which induces generation of T-cells
Antigen supplies to immunocompetent cells
Local production of angiotensin-converting enzyme (ACE)
Promotion of production of adhesion molecules that participate in the inflammatory reaction

3. Detection of biochemical changes in blood and maintenance of homeostasis

Recognition of variations of pH and oxygen and CO_2 concentration, participating in this way in vascular homeostasis

4. Autocrine function

Release of vasoactive substances that regulate vascular tone:
◆ Nitric oxide, prostacyclin
◆ Endothelin, thromboxane
◆ Angiotensin-I, angiotensin-II, angiotensin (1-7)

5. Control of growth and proliferation

Induction of production of vascular smooth muscle promoters
Induction of production of vascular smooth muscle inhibitors
Induction of adhesion molecules for blood cells

6. Hemostatic function

Insurance of blood fluidity
Thromboresistant activity through anticoagulant, fibrinolytic, and platelet antiaggregation properties
Promotion of the production of procoagulant and anticoagulant substances: PGI_2, endothelin I, fibronectin, tissue-type plasminogen activator, heparin and PAI-I (plasminogen activator inhibitor-I)

Vascular Endothelial Function[3,4,67,105]

Vasomotor Tone

Vasodilators

Nitric oxide (NO)
Prostacyclin (PGI_2)
Endothelium-derived hyperpo-
    larizing factor (EDHF)
Bradykinin (BK)
Serotonin (S)
Histamine (H)
Substance P (SP)
Angiotensin (1-7) (Ang 1-7)
C-type natriuretic peptide
    (CNP)
Adrenomedullin (AM)
Angiotensin (1-9) (Ang 1-9)
Atrial natriuretic peptide (ANP)
Brain natriuretic peptide (BNP)
DNP

Vasoconstrictors

Angiotensin-II (Ang-II)
Endothelin-1 (ET-1)
Angiotensin-I (Ang-I)
Angiotensin-III (Ang-III)
Thrombin
Endoperoxides
Prostaglandin 2 (PG-2)
Prostaglandin H_2 (PG-H_2)
Thromboxane A_2 (TxA_2)
Serotonin (S)
Arachidonic acid (AA)
Nicotine
Angiotensin-IV (Ang-IV)
Platelet-derived growth factor
    (PDGF)

Discussion

A balance of vasodilators and vasocontrictors will determine vascular tone. NO and PGI_2 are the primary vasodilators that relax
vascular smooth muscle, and reduce systemic vascular resistance
and BP. Ang II and ET-1 are the predominant vasoconstrictors that
constrict VSM, increase SVR, and elevate BP.

Growth (VSM)

Growth Inhibitors

Nitric oxide (NO)
Transforming growth factor β (TGF-β)
Heparin-like molecules (HLMs) (HS)
Bradykinin (BK)
Prostacyclin (PGI$_2$)
Angiotensin (1-7 (Ang 1-7)
Heparin sulfate (HS)
Heparin-like glycosaminogly-cans (GAGs)
Thrombospondin

Growth Promoters

Platelet-derived growth factor (PDGF)
Basic fibroblast growth factor (βFGF)
Insulin-like growth factor-1 (IGF-1)
Endothelin 1 (ET-1)
Angiotensin-II (Ang-II)
Angiotensin-III (Ang-III)
Angiotensin-IV (Ang-IV)
Vascular endothelial growth factor (VEGF)

Vascular Endothelial Function[3,4,67,105]

Thrombosis

Anti-Thrombotic

Prostacyclin (PGI2)
Nitric oxide (NO)
Thrombomodulin (TBM)
Heparin-like proteoglycans
(HLP)
Ecto-ADPase (CD 39)
Tissue plasminogen activator
(tPA)
Urokinase (UK)

Pro-Thrombotic

Plasminogen activator
inhibitor-1 (PAI-1)
Thromboxane A2 (TxA2)
Tissue factor (TF)
von Willebrand factor (vWF)
Platelet-activating factor (PAF)

Inflammation

Anti-Inflammatory

Nitric oxide (NO/EDRF)
Bradykinin (BK)
Prostacyclin (PGI2)
Anti-oxidant enzymes (SOD,
GTP)
Complement regulatory factors
(CRFs)
Kininase-II

Pro-Inflammatory

Leukocyte recruitment
Endothelial leukocyte adhesion
molecules (ELAMs)
Selectins
Intercellular adhesion mole-
cules (ICAMs)
Vascular adhesion molecules
(VCAMs)
Chemoattractants
Chemoactivators
Interleukin-8 (IL-8)
Monocyte chemoattractant pro-
tein-1 (MCP-1)
Platelet-activating factor (PAF)
Cytokines (M-CSF, GM-CSF)
Chemokines

Vascular Endothelial Function[3,4,67,105]

Oxidative Stress/REDOX

Antioxidant

Nitric oxide (NO)
Bradykinin (BK)
COX-1, COX-2
Mn SOD, Cu/Zn SOD

Oxidant

Angiotensin-II (Ang-II)
Endothelin-1 (ET-1)
Cytokines
Growth factors

Selective Permeability Barrier

Tight and gap functions
Junctional proteins
Endocytic receptors
Cell surface glycocalix

Endothelium-dependent Responses[5]

(not present in all blood vessels)

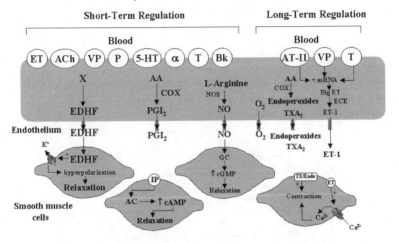

Activation of endothelial receptors can stimulate NO synthase [NOS, which produces nitric oxide (NO)], and cyclooxygenase [COX, which produces prostacyclin (PGI$_2$) from arachidonic acid (AA)] and can lead to the release of endothelium-derived hyperpolarizing factor (EDHF). NO causes relaxation by activating the formation of cyclic GMP (cGMP) from guanosine triphosphate (GTP) by soluble guanylate cyclase (GC). Prostacyclin (PGI$_2$) causes relaxation by activating adenylate cyclase (AC) leading to the formation of cyclic AMP (cAMP). EDHF causes hyperpolarization and relaxation by opening K$^+$ channels. Any increase in cytosolic calcium (including that induced by the calcium ionophore A23187) causes the release of relaxing factors. In certain blood vessels, contracting substances can be released from the endothelial cells, which include superoxide anions (O$_2^-$), thromboxane A$_2$ (TXA$_2$), endoperoxides, and possibly endothelin-1 (ET-1). Thromboxane A$_2$ and endoperoxides activate specific receptors (TX/Endo) on the vascular smooth muscle, as does ET1 (ET). Such activation causes an increase in intracellular Ca^{2+}, leading to contraction. The production of ET-1 [catalyzed by endothelin-converting enzyme (ECE)] can be augmented by angiotensin II (ATII), vasopressin (VP), or thrombin (T). The neurohumoral mediators that cause the release of endothelium-derived relaxing factors (and sometimes contracting factors) through activation of specific endothelial receptors (circles) include: acetylcholine (ACh), adenosine diphosphate (P), bradykinin (BK), endothelin (ET), adrenaline (α), serotonin (5HT), thrombin (T), and vasopressin (VP).

Control Endothelial Cell[5]

Postulated signal transduction processes in a normal endothelial cell are shown. Activation of the cell causes the release of EDRF-NO, which has important protective effects in the vascular wall.

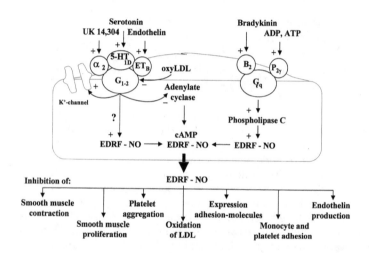

α, alpha-adrenergic; 5-HT, serotonin receptor; ET, endothelin receptors; B, bradykinin receptor; P, purinoceptor; G, coupling proteins; cAMP, cyclic adenosine monophosphate; EDRF, endothelium-derived relaxing factor; NO, nitric oxide; LDL, low-density lipoprotein; UK, urokinase; K+, potassium; +, activation; −, inhibition. (Modified from reference 24).

Endothelium-derived Vasoactive Substances[6]

Various blood- and platelet-derived substances can activate specific receptors (open circles) on the endothelial membrane to release relaxing factors such as nitric oxide (NO), prostacyclin (PGI_2), and endothelium-derived hyperpolarizing factor (EDHF). Other contracting factors are released, such as endothelin-1 (ET-1), angiotensin (Ang), and thromboxane A_2 (TXA_2), as well as prostaglandin H_2 (PGH_2).

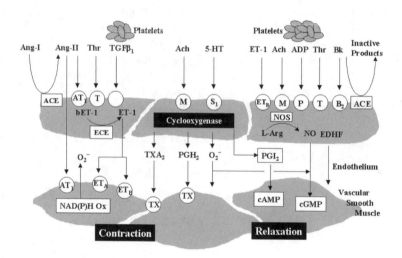

O_2^-, superoxide; Thr, thrombin; TGF-β1, transforming growth factor-β1; Ach, acetylcholine; 5-HT, serotonin; Bk, bradykinin; ACE, angiotensin-converting enzyme; ECE, endothelin-converting enzyme; eNOS, endothelial nitric oxide synthase; L-Arg, L-arginine; NO, nitric oxide; AT_1, angiotensin I receptor.

Summary
Endothelial Function

The primary function of the endothelium is to maintain vascular homeostasis. The strategic anatomical location of the endothelium between the lumen and the vascular smooth muscle modulates vasomotor tone, growth, thrombosis, inflammation, and oxidative stress. The relative balance of these mediators determines vascular function and structure and thus vascular health or disease:

Vasoconstrictors	vs.	Vasodilators
Growth Promoters	vs.	Growth Inhibitors
Prothrombotic	vs.	Antithrombotic
Inflammatory	vs.	Antiinflammatory
Oxidant	vs.	Antioxidant
Permeable	vs.	Nonpermeable

Complex interactive pathways, receptor activation, and signal transduction are part of the *endothelial activation* process.

Chapter 5
Endothelial Vasodilators

Nitric Oxide (NO): Definition[4,5,8,9,10]

Involved in numerous biologic processes

Most powerful endogenous vasodilator. Basal vascular tone produced and released both tonically and under stimulation

Inhibits atherosclerotic process

Also known as endothelium-derived relaxing factor or EDRF (EDRF is really NO and more)

Synthesized by nitric oxide synthase (NOS) in:
  Endothelium (eNOS)
  Platelets
  Macrophages
  Neurons
  Vascular smooth muscle cells (VSMCs)

Women produce more NO than men

Short $T^1/_2$ (seconds); increased with binding to albumin (nitrosylation)

Nitric Oxide and Endothelium-Derived Relaxing Factor[98,107]

Endothelium-derived relaxing factor (EDRF) includes:
  NO
  SNO (S-nitrothiols)
  Metal–NO complexes
  S-Nitrosoglutathione

Clinical importance
  Develop exogenous arterial EDRF/NO donors to stimulate these endogenous compounds to reduce hypertension and atherosclerosis.

Nitric Oxide: Mechanism[98,107]

NO interacts with substances to produce **vasodilation**
Metal-containing proteins
Thiol proteins

NO + HEME in sGC → ↑ cGMP
NO + thiol in K^+ channels → open K^+ channels

VSMC myogenic contraction may be balance of NO and HETE (hydroxy-eicosatetraenoic acid)
HETE from arachidonic acid (AA) via P450 4A in VSMC
HETE inhibits K^+ channels
HETE production inhibited by NO

---

sGC, soluble guanyl cyclase; cGMP, cyclic guanosine monophosphate.

Biologic Functions[101]

➤ Neurotransmission

➤ Cardiovascular control

➤ Atherosclerosis

➤ Cell growth and apoptosis

➤ Inflammation and infection

➤ Renal function:
Glomerular and renal hemodynamics
Renin release
SNS transmission
Sodium and water excretion
Tubuloglomerular feedback

Major Cardiovascular Effects[107]

Vasodilation (VSMC): ↑ cGMP, ↑ cAMP (secondary), ↓ ET-1
Anti-atherosclerotic: Modulates leukocyte-vessel wall interaction
                 ↑ cGMP, ↓ CAM, ↓ chemokines
Antiplatelet: ↑ cGMP, ↑ cAMP, ↑ PGI$_2$, ↑ tPA
Antigrowth: VSM hypertrophy, proliferation, migration
Antioxidant: ↓ O$_2^-$, ↓ oxLDL

VSMC, vascular smooth muscle cell; cGMP, cyclic guanosine monophosphate; cAMP, cyclic adenosine monophosphate; ET-1, endothelin-1; CAM, cell adhesion molecule; PGI$_2$, prostacyclin; tPA, tissue-type plasminogen activator; O$_2^-$, superoxide anion; oxLDL, oxidized LDL cholesterol.

Antiatherosclerotic Properties of NO Produced by the Vascular Endothelium[9]

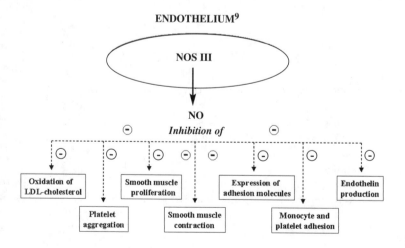

ENDOTHELIUM[9]

NOS III

NO

⊖   *Inhibition of*   ⊖

| Oxidation of LDL-cholesterol | Smooth muscle proliferation | Expression of adhesion molecules | Endothelin production |

| Platelet aggregation | Smooth muscle contraction | Monocyte and platelet adhesion |

Biological Effects of NO in the Cardiovascular System[27,97]

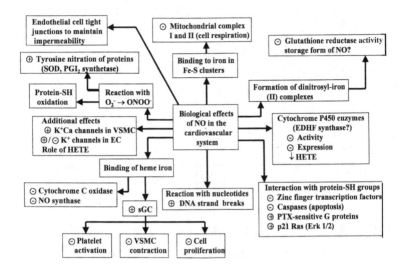

Cardioprotection and Drugs[98]

NO is partly responsible for cardioprotective effects of:

Nitroglycerin

Nitroprusside

Angiotensin-converting enzyme inhibitors (ACEIs)

Estrogens

Statins

Calcium channel blockers (CCBs)

Angiotensin receptor blockers (ARBs)

Renal Effects[101]

Schematic summary of the mechanisms resulting in sustained hypertension due to nitric oxide synthase (NOS) inhibition or deficiency. ATPase; adenosine triphospatase; GFR; glomerular filtration rate; TGF, tubuloglomerular feedback; Kf, filtration fraction.

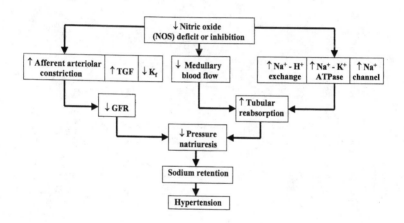

NO Relationship with pGC/sGC, cGMP, cAMP, ANF, and PGI$_2$[1,100]

Nitric oxide difuses into the VSMC and stimulates sGC, which converts GTP into cGMP. cGMP inhibits PDE, which increases cAMP levels. PGI$_2$ also increases cAMP via AC, and ANF increases pGC and thus increases cGMP. Both **cGMP** and **cAMP** cause **VSM relaxation**.

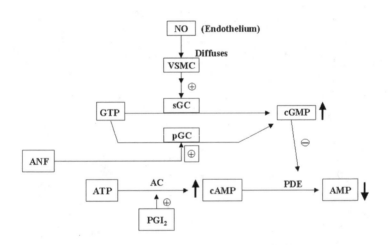

NO, nitric oxide; VSMC, vascular smooth muscle cell; sGC, soluble guanyl cyclase; pGC, particulate guanyl cyclase; GTP, guanosine triphosphate; cGMP, cyclic guanosine monophosphate; ANF, atrial natriuretic factor; ATP, adenosine triphosphate; AC, adenyl cyclase; PGI$_2$, prostacyclin; cAMP, cyclic adenosine monophosphate; PDE, phosphodiesterase; AMP, adenosine monophosphate.

NO Relationship with cAMP, cGMP, PGI$_2$, COX, and ANF[5]

Interaction between nitric oxide (NO) and the catabolism of cyclic adenosine monophosphate (cAMP).

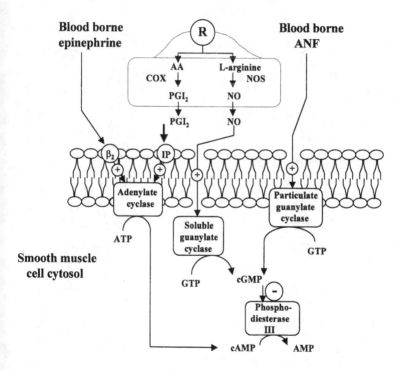

R, cell membrane receptor; AA, arachidonic acid; PGI$_2$, prostacyclin; COX, cyclooxygenase; NOS, nitric oxide synthase; ANF, atrial natriuretic factor; β_2, beta$_2$-adrenergic receptor; IP, prostacyclin receptor; cGMP, cyclic guanosine monophosphate; cAMP, cyclic adenosine monophosphate; ATP, adenosine triphosphate; GTP, guanosine triphosphate; +, activation; –, inhibition.

Nitric Oxide Metabolic Pathways: Overview[102,107]

L-arginine is the precursor for NO via NOS. It also may be metabolized to L-ornithine or Agmatine, which may reduce blood pressure through stimulation of the imidazoline receptor on endothelial cells.

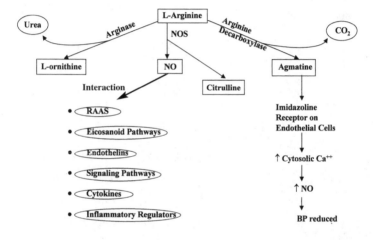

Nitric Oxide Pathways[1,100,101,107]
Metabolic Products, Cofactors, ADMA

ADMA (asymmetric dimethylarginine) can inhibit NO and neutralize its vascular protective effects. ADMA is increased in patients with hypertension and hyperlipidemia. Adequate substrate, cosubstrates, and cofactors must be avilable for NO production. Adequate DDAH (dimethylarginine dimethylaminohydrolase) must be present to break down ADMA.

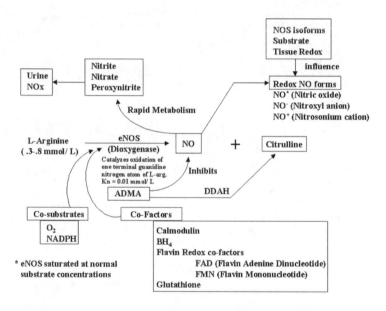

NO, nitric oxide; ADMA, asymmetric dimethyl arginine; DDAH, dimethylarginine dimethylaminohydrolase; BH_4, tetrahydrobiopterin; NADPH, reduced nicotinamide adenine dinucleotide phosphate; FAD, flavin adenine dinucleotide; FMN, flavin mononucleotide.

Nitric Oxide Synthesis:
Stimulant Pathways[9,27,100,101,102,107]

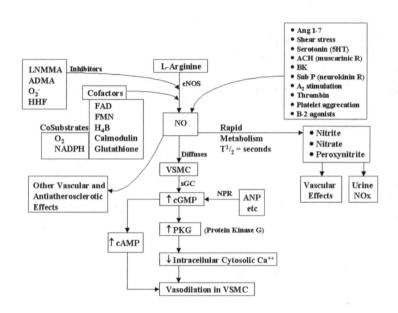

HHF = Hepatic Hypertensive Factor
ANP = Atrial Natriuretic Peptide

NO, L-NMMA Stimulant Pathways[9]

Mechanisms of endothelium-dependent vasodilation: the L-arginine/nitric oxide (NO) pathway. Endothelial NO synthase (NOS III) can be stimulated by acetylcholine through the muscarinic receptor. The signal transduction pathway includes the receptor Gi complex and the Ca^{2+}/calmodulin pathway. Substance P stimulates a different receptor, bradykinin uses a different receptor/G-protein complex and β_2-agonists can stimulate NOS III independently of the Ca^{2+}/calmodulin pathway. NOS III can be blocked by the L-arginine analogue NG-monomethyl-L-arginine (L-NMMA). NO is produced in the presence of the NOS-cofactor tetrahydrobiopterin (BH_4). NO stimulates soluble guanylate cyclase to produce cyclic guanosine 5'-monophosphate (GMP), which induces endothelium-dependent vasodilation in the smooth muscle cell.

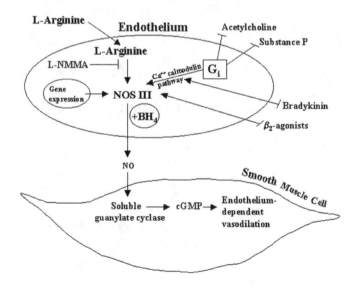

ADMA and DDAH[28,100]

ADMA (Asymmetric Dimethylargininine)

➤ Autocrine regulator of eNOS
➤ Inhibits eNOS and reduces NO (competitive substrate)
➤ Elevated in hypertensive children and young adults
➤ Elevated in DM, CRI, smokers, HBP, HLP, elderly, atherosclerosis
➤ VCAM and VWF positively correlate with increased ADMA
➤ Levels of ADMA (endothelial > plasma levels)

Normal	1.0 ± 0.1 µmol/L
HLP	2.2 ± 0.2 µmol/L
HBP	2.2 ± 0.2 µmol/L
Elderly with AS	2.5 ± 3.5 µmol/L

oxLDL ⟶ ↑ ADMA ⟶ Citrulline

Methionine (homocysteine) ⟶ (to ↑ ADMA)   DDAH

eNOS + ADMA → O_2- → NFκB activation → ↑ MCP-1

DDAH (Dimethylarginine Dimethylaminohydrolase)

➤ Inhibited by: oxLDL, PPAR, cytokines (TNF-α)
➤ Stimulated by: retinoic acid

VCAM, vascular cell adhesion molecule; vWF, von Willebrand factor; NFκB, nuclear factor kappa B; MCP-1, monocyte chemoattractant protein-1; PPAR, peroxisome proliferator-activated receptor; TNF-α, tumor necrosis factor-alpha; eNOS, endothelial nitric oxide synthase.

NO and ADMA[9]

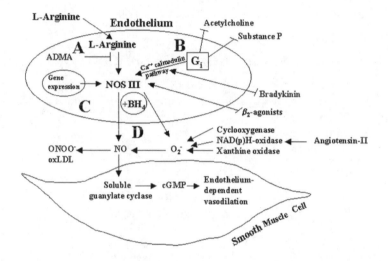

Potential mechanisms that may disturb endothelial NO bioavailability: Diminished NO synthesis due to: (a) substrate deficiency or/and competitive inhibition of endothelial NO synthase (NOS III) by endogenous NGNG-dimethyl-L-arginine (ADMA); (b) disturbances in signal transduction related to the receptor/G-protein complex or the Ca^{2+}/calmodulin pathway; (c) reduced activity of NOS III; or (d) enhanced breakdown of NO due to enhanced superoxide production.

Superoxide may be generated by NOS III itself (especially if the cofactor tetrahydrobiopterin (BH_4) is depleted), xanthine oxidases, the cyclooxygenase pathway or NAD(P)H-driven oxidases which can be stimulated by angiotensin-II via AT_1 receptors. Superoxide anion scavenges NO to produce peroxynitrite ($ONOO^-$). Superoxide can also lead to the formation of oxidized low density lipoprotein (oxLDL).

Nitric Oxide Synthase (NOS)[27,97–100]

There are three isoforms of NOS:

1. Neuronal NOS (nNOS or NOS-I)
2. Inducible NOS (iNOS or NOS-II)
3. Endothelial NOS (eNOS, ENDO, or NOS-III)

Neuronal NOS (nNOS or NOS-I)

➢ Vasomotor centers CNS and PNS
➢ Neuronal networks adventitial surfaces blood vessels (VSMC, myocytes)
➢ Intracardiac neurons
➢ Gene located on chromosome 12q24.2

Inducible NOS (iNOS, NOS-II)
(Macrophage-Immune NOS)

➢ Calcium-dependent
➢ Located in developing fetus, ductus arteriosus endothelium and vascular smooth muscle
➢ Increased in injury, inflammation, infection, congestive heart failure
➢ Increased by homocysteine
➢ Secondary location in endotoxin and cytokinase treated neutrophils, hepatocytes, endothelial cells, myocardium
➢ Gene located on chromosome 17cen-q11.2
➢ Cytokine-induced
➢ Long-term superior responses

Endothelial NOS (eNOS, ENDO, NOS-III)

➤ Constitutively expressed membrane-bound enzyme on endothelium vascular cells
➤ Localized to Golgi appartus, plasmalemma, caveolae (contain signal transducers like G proteins, tyrosine kinases, serine kinases)
➤ Both Ca^{2+}-calmodulin-dependent and Ca^{2+}-independent
➤ Regulation of activity:
  Intracellular Ca^{2+}
  Intracellular pH
  Interaction with caveolin-1
  Interaction with membrane phospholipids
  Reversible N-terminal palmitoylation of enzyme
  Phosphorylation
  Heat shock protein-90 (HSP-90)
  Transcription factors (activator protein-1 [AP-1]), NF-κB)
  Estrogen
  Vascular endothelial growth factor (VEGF)
  Insulin
  Shear stress
➤ Located on:
  Endothelial cells of large arteries and resistance vessels
  Capillaries and veins
  Endocardial cells
  Cardiac myocytes
  Cardiac pacemaker cells
  Platelets
  Mononucelar cells
  Corpus cavenosum sinusoids
➤ eNOS generates in a short-term response:
  NO
  O_2^- (if deficient in BH_4 or L-arginine)
➤ Gene located on chromosome 7q35-36
➤ Polymorphism with variable number of tandem repeats (VNTR) at intron 4 contributes to fasting NOx in healthy individual. This is associated with **hypertension** and **CHD**.

NO and Free Radicals: ROS, O_2^-, $OH^{\bullet 5}$

Interactions between nitric oxide (NO) and superoxide anions (O_2^-). Superoxide anions cause contraction of vascular smooth muscle by scavenging endothelium-derived NO and by activating the production of vasoconstrictor prostaglandins in the vascular smooth muscle cells, presumably after transformation to hydroxyl radicals ($OH^{\bullet}$).

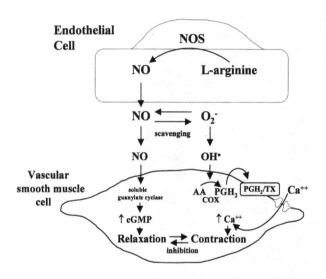

AA, arachidonic acid; COX, cyclooxygenase; cGMP, cyclic guanosine monophosphate; NOS, nitric oxide synthase; PGH_2, endoperoxide; TX, thromboxane; Ca^{++}, calcium.

Nitric Oxide: Reduced Bioactivity

Early Endothelial Dysfunction[3,4,9,100]

➤ **Decreased Production of NO**

L-arginine substrate deficiency (age, HBP, HLP)

ADMA competitive inhibition of eNOS (HBP, HLP, CVD)

Reduced eNOS activity (oxLDL, cytokines, ROS)

Reduced CAT-1 and reduced BH_4

Increased arginase or arginase decarboxylase activity

Renal excretion of L-arginine

➤ **HEME Degradation of NO**

HEME-mediated oxidation–oxyhemoglobin

ROS (O_2^-) and eNOS-III $\rightarrow O_2^-$ production

BH_4 depletion (tetrahydrobiopterin) (O_2^-)

Xanthine oxidases

Cyclooxygenase pathway (EDCF, HETE, O_2^-, ET-1)

Ang-II, NAD(P)H oxidases, O_2^- via AT1R upregulation
(LDL also upregulates AT_1R)

NOS alteration

➤ **Disturbed Receptor and/or Signal Transduction**

Surface receptor (shear stress, MR, MK-1R, B2R)

G protein complex $(G_1$ and $G_2)$ (HLP, HBP?)

Ca^{2+}/ calmodulin pathway (HBP, ? HLP)

➤ **Disruption of Cellular Environment**

"AGE" products

Homocysteine

Folate, B_6, B_{12} deficiency

Possible Mechanisms of Reduced Endothelium-derived NO Activity[100]

Disruption of normal NO signaling mechanisms
 Disruption of cell surface receptors (shear stress-sensing glyco-
 proteins, muscarinic receptors, neurokinin 1 and B_2 receptors)
 Inhibition of endothelium Ca^{2+} influx, or binding to calmodulin

Reduced availability of substrate
 Dietary arginine deficiency
 Reduced activity/expression of arginase or arginine decarboxylase
 Reduced activity of arginosuccinate synthase
 Compartmentalization of arginine, CAT-1 and NOS
 Decreased renal tubular reuptake of L-arginine
 Antagonism of NOS

Overproduction of ADMA or other competitive inhibitor of NOS
 Decreased activity/expression of DDAH
 Inhibition by endogenous NO
 Inhibition by exogenous NO donors

Alterations in NOS
 Reduced expression
 Reduced dimerization
 Aberrant palmitoylation, myristolation, or phosphorylation

Decreased affinity of L-arginine for NOS
 Reduced generation of tetrahydrobiopterin

Increased degradation of NO
 Increased generation of superoxide and hydrogen peroxide

Disruption of cellular environment of NOS
 Advanced glycosylation end-products
 Hyperhomocysteinemia, homocystinuria
 Folate deficiency

NO, nitric oxide; CAT, cationic amino acid transporter; NOS, nitric oxide synthase; ADMA, asymmetric dimethylarginine; DDAH, dimethylarginine dimethylaminohydrolase; B_2, bradykinin type 2 receptor.

Nitric Oxide and Hypertension[97]

➢ Reduced NO in hypertension contributes to endothelial dysfunction (ED)
➢ ED may be primary or secondary
➢ Acute hypertension with SBP > 200 mmHg for 15 min disrupts endothelial junction and increases ED
➢ Increased superoxide anion (O_2^-) production in hypertension
➢ NO neutralizes O_2^-
➢ Aging and hypertension have decreased soluble guanadyl cyclase (sGC) expression and its NO-dependent activation in aortic tissue[16]
➢ Acetylcholine (ACh) and substance P response is also abnormal in hypertension
➢ In CHD: ACh → vasoconstricts
               Substance P response is normal

Nitric Oxide and Hypertension
(NO and O_2^- and Peroxynitrite)[3,97]

Superoxide anion (O_2^-) sources
    NADH oxidase
    eNOS + ADMA
    Cyclooxygenase
    Cytochrome P450
    Lysophosphatidylcholine (LPC) via PKC

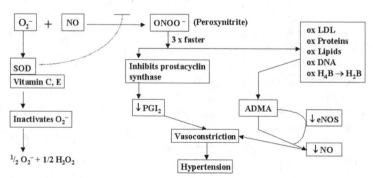

SOD, superoxide dismutase; PGI_2, prostacyclin; ADMA, asymmetric dimethyl arginine; eNOS, endothelial nitric oxide synthase; ox H_4B, oxidized tetrahydrobiopterin.

Nitric Oxide and Hypertension Therapeutic Relationships[9,100]

L-arginine (competitive inhibitor of ADMA) improves endothelial vasodilation (EDV) in:

    Hyperlipidemia (HLP)

    Congestive heart failure (CHF)

    Peripheral vascular disease (PVD)

    Hypertension (HBP) (controversial)

    Insulin-dependent diabetes mellitus
      (IDDM) (controversial)

Nitroglycerin and nitroprusside are NO donors

Increased NO levels with some antihypertensive drugs

ACEIs	($\uparrow$ BK [bradykinin] $\rightarrow$ $\uparrow$ NO + $\downarrow$ O_2^-)
CCBs	($\uparrow$ NO, $\downarrow$ ROS [reactive oxygen species])
ARBs	($\uparrow$ BK, $\uparrow$ NO, $\downarrow$ ROS)

NO also increased by:

Statins	
Estrogens	($\uparrow$ eNOS)
Exercise	($\uparrow$ shear stress $\rightarrow$ $\uparrow$ eNOS)
H_4B	($\uparrow$ eNOS, $\downarrow$ H_4B in HLP)
Antioxidants	($\downarrow$ O_2^-, $\downarrow$ ROS)
ASA	($\uparrow$ iNOS in VSMC, $\downarrow$ platelet activity)

Discussion

Several antihypertensive drugs increase NO bioavailibility through various mechanisms:

◆ ACEIs increase BK levels, which increase NO through the BK receptor. They also reduce ROS such as superoxide anion (O_2^-), which increases NO availability.

◆ ARBs also increase BK levels and decrease ROS and O_2^-, both of which increase NO bioavailibility.

◆ CCBs increase NO primarily through an antioxidant effect, which reduces ROS.

Other compounds such as statins, estrogen, tetrahydrobiopterin (H_4B), ASA, and antioxidants increase NO bioavailibility.

Hypertension and Hyperlipidemia[9]

Role of Ang-II, LDL, and AT$_1$R

Relationship between hypertension and hyperlipidemia and why statins may decrease BP

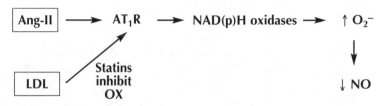

Statins reduce formation of oxidized LDL, which reduces O_2^- and elevates NO. This reduces BP, improves ED, and has a vascular protective effect.
ACEIs and ARBs reduce stimulation of AT$_1$R and also increase NO.

Potential Differences in Proposed Mechanism for Impaired Nitric Oxide (NO) Bioavailability Between Arterial Hypertension and Hypercholesterolemia[9]

	Arterial Hypertension	Hypercholes-terolemia
NO bioavailability	↓	↓
Basal NO release	↓	Ø
Stimulated NO release	↓	↓
Diminished NO synthesis		
L-arginine substrate deficiency	Ø	+
ADMA	?	+
Muscarinic receptor	Ø	Ø
Receptor-Gi complex	Ø	+
Ca^{2+}/calmodulin pathway	+	Ø
NOS activity	?	(+)
Enhanced NO breakdown		
Superoxide production	+	+
Xanthine oxidase	Ø	+
Cyclooxygenase pathway	+	?
NOS-III/BH$_4$ depletion	?	+
Angiotensin-II/NAD(P)H-oxidases	?	+

+, Evidence for the potential mechanism; Ø, no evidence for the potential mechanism; ?, not investigated, ADAM, NGNG-dimethyl-L-arginine.

Summary Functions of NO[4,5,8–10,28,98]

1. Most powerful endogenous vasodilator[4,9] (↓ VSMC contraction)
2. Maintains basal vascular tone[4]
3. Inhibits migration of VSMC[4,9]
4. Inhibits leukocyte adhesion to endothelium[4,9]
5. Inhibits platelet aggregation and granule secretion[28]
6. Major role in architecture and remodeling of blood vessels[4]
7. Inhibits VSMC proliferation[5,9]
8. Inhibits oxidation of LDL[5,9]
9. Inhibits ET-1 production[5,9] and action[5]
   ◆ NO inhibits expression of mRNA for ET-1 production
   ◆ NO inhibits action of ET-1 at ET-A receptor
10. Promotes apoptosis[8]
11. Protects against target organ damage (left ventricular hypertrophy [LVH], renal, cardiac, cerebral, etc.)[8]
12. Decreases endothelial permeability[9]
13. Inhibits expression of adhesion molecules (CAMs)[9]
14. Suppresses TNFα-induced NF-κB activation in endothelium[10]
15. Renal vasodilation with diuresis and natriuresis[12]
16. Inhibits aldosterone secretion in zona glomerulosa of adrenal gland[21]
17. Inhibits platelet–endothelium denuded vessel wall interaction[28]
18. Inhibits platelet adhesion to endothelial cell monolayers[28]
19. Inhibits proinflammatory cytokines[28]
20. Modulates baroreceptor reflexes[98]

Endothelium Vasodilators

◆ Bradykinin (BK)
◆ Prostacyclin (PGI$_2$)
◆ Endothelium-dependent hyperpolarizing factor (EDHF)
◆ Angiotensin-(1-7) [Ang-(1-7)]
◆ Angiotensin-(1-9) [Ang-(1-9)]
◆ Serotonin (variable → VC or VD)
◆ Histamine
◆ Substance P
◆ C-type natriuretic peptide (CNP) and ANP, BNP, DNP
◆ Adrenomedullin (AM)

Bradykinin[4,23]

1. Direct potent vasodilator

2. Stimulates release of NO (primary vasodilation action)

3. Stimulates release of EDHF

4. Promotes production of t-PA

5. Inhibits platelet aggregation via release of NO and Prostacyclin

6. Stimulates release of prostacyclin (PGI$_2$)

7. Direct stimulation of bradykinin-2 receptor improves insulin-mediated glucose transport and decreases insulin resistance (Glut 1-4)

8. Bradykinin is degraded by:

    Angiotensin-converting enzyme (ACE)

    Neutral endopeptidase (NEP)

    Endothelin-converting enzyme (ECE)

    Metalloendopeptidase thermolysin-like enzymes
       (EP 24.15 and EP 24.16)

    Carboxypeptidases

    Aminopeptidases

Prostacyclin (PGI$_2$)[1,5]

1. Fatty acid derivative synthesized from arachidonic acid
2. Induces or activates adenylate cyclase with:
   An increased cAMP in VSMC and platelets resulting in vasodilation and platelet aggregation reduction and reduced VSMC growth
3. Formed mainly in intima
4. Note: COX-2 inhibitors may decrease PGI$_2$ and decrease cAMP with resultant vasoconstriction and increased BP

Endothelium-dependent Hyperpolarizing Factor (EDHF)[27]

1. EDHF hyperpolarizes VSMC by opening K$^+$ channels
2. EDHF is either:
   A. Cytochrome P-450 derived arachidonic acid metabolite
   B. Potassium ion

Discussion

BK levels are increased by ACEIs and ARBs. ACEIs inhibit the ACE (kininase) that breaks down BK; thus BK increases. ACEIs also inhibit the breakdown of substance P. Accumulation of BK and substance P contributes to the relative high incidence of cough with use of ACEIs (15-20%) compared to ARBs. ARBs increase BK via effects on the AT$_2$ receptor and kinogenase. Substance P is not affected, and thus cough is rare with ARBs.

Kinin System[4,23]

Bradykinin stimulates the B_2R (bradykinin 2 receptor), which produces favorable vascular effects that reduce blood pressure, thrombotic potential, and glucose. Both ACEIs and ARBs increase bradykinin levels.

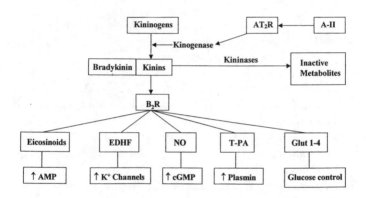

AT_2R, angiotensin-II receptor; A-II, angiotensin-II; B_2R, bradykinin-2 receptor; EDHF, endothelium-dependent hyperpolarizing factor; NO, nitric oxide; tPA, tissue-type plasminogen activator; AMP, adenosine monophosphate; K+, potassium; cGMP, cyclic guanosine monophosphate; Glut 1-4, glucose 1-4 receptor.

Angiotensin-(1-7)[4,67]

1. Aminoterminal heptapeptide
2. Produced in many different tissues

3.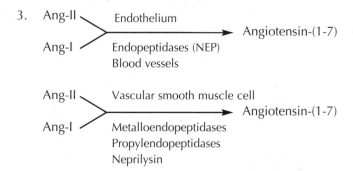

4. Vasodilator via NO and BK productions and release
5. Opposes Ang-II on growth and reactivity of blood vessels
6. NO vasoconstriction, NO aldosterone release, NO antiduretic hormone release, NO induction of noradrenergic neurotransmission
7. Endopeptidases also break down ET-1 (endothelin)
8. Role of Ang-(1-7)
   Potent vasodilator, natriuretics/diuretics
   Blocks VSMC proliferation and VSMC contraction
   ↑ NO + ↑ BK
   ↑ PGI_2
   Inhibits ACE
9. Mediated via AT_{1-7} receptor, **not** AT_1 or AT_2 receptors
10. ACEIs increase angiotensin-(1-7) by 5–50 x in tissue and circulation, as well as increase Ang-I
11. Angiotensin-(1-7) is both a substrate and an inhibitor of ACE
12. ARBs increase Ang-II by 8-10 x

Actions of Angiotensin-(1-7)[104]

Actions Different from Those of Angotensin-II

Cardiovascular System
Hypotension
Endothelium-dependent vasodilation
Potentiation of the hypotensive effects of bradykinin
Inhibition of rat aortic smooth muscle cell growth
Increased baroreflex control of heart rate

Kidney
Antidiuresis in water-loaded rats
Natriuresis, diuresis, and increase in glomerular filtration rate in isolated perfused rat kidney, spontaneously hypertensive rats, and anesthetized Wistar rats

Actions Similar to and Approximately Equipotent to Those of Angiotensin-II

General
Stimulation of prostaglandin production in rabbit isolated vasa deferentia, rat smooth muscle cells, human astrocytes, and C6 glioma cells

Nervous System
Stimulation of vasopressin release
Stimulation of substance P release from rat hypothalamus
Dilatation of piglet pial arterioles
Stimulation of psychotropic activity

Cardiovascular System
Cardiovascuclar effects of microinjection into the medulla of rats
Stimulation of proliferation of human cardia fibroblasts
Coronary vasoconstriction and facilitation of reperfusion arrhythmias
Stimulation of 3H-norepinephrine release from rat atria
Stimulation of nitric oxide production by dog coronary vessels

Kidney
Stimulation of phospholipase activity and transcellular sodium flux in renal proximal tubule cells

48

Endothelium Vasodilators: Summary

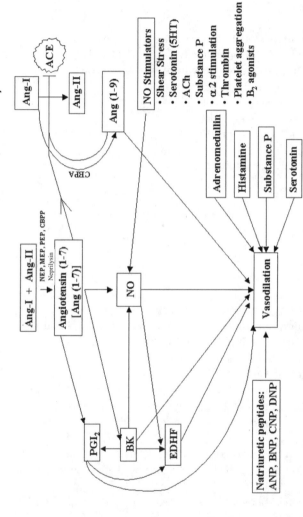

Ang I=angiotensin I, Ang II=angiotensin II, NEP= neutral endopeptidases, MEP= metalloendopeptidases, PEP= propylendopeptidases, CBPP= carboxyl B proteopeptidase, CBPA= carboxyl A proteopeptidase, ANG (1-9)= angiotensin (1-9), PGI_2= prostacyclin, BK= bradykinin, EDHF= endothelial hyperpolarizing factor, NO= nitric oxide, Ach= acetylcholine.

Discussion

The various vasodilators relax VSM through numerous pathways. Angiotensin-(1-7) [Ang-(1-7)] accumulates in the presence of ACEI and it stimulates production of PGI_2, BK, NO, Ang-(1-9) and indirectly EDHF, all causing vasodilation. Alternate enzymatic pathways (NEP, MEP, PEP, CBPP, neprilysin, CBPA) contribute to the formation of Ang-(1-7) and Ang-(1-9).

The natriuretic peptides adrenomedullin, histamine, substance P, and serotonin cause direct vasodilation via separate mechanisms. The NO stimulators directly increase NO production.

Summary
Endothelial Vasodilators:
Nitric Oxide and Other Vasodilators

The most prominent and important vasodilator is nitric oxide (NO). NO has numerous favorable cardiovascular effects, including vasodilation, antiatherosclerotic, antiplatelet, anti-growth, and antioxidants. Many drugs such as ARBs, ACEIs, CCBs, and statins increase NO bioavailibility, which accounts for much of their favorable effects on the vascular system.

Other vasodilators contribute to vascular tone and effects that are similar to NO. These include BK, PGI_2, EDHF, Ang-(1-7), Ang-(1-9), AM, and natriuretic peptides.

Chapter 6
Endothelium Vasoconstrictors[4]

1. Endothelin (ET-1)

2. Angiotensins
   A. Angiotensin-I (Ang-I)
   B. Angiotensin-II (Ang-II)
   C. Angiotensin-III (Ang-III)
   D. Angiotensin-IV (Ang-IV)
   E. Angiotensin-X (Ang-X) (unknown)

3. Aldosterone

4. Cycloxygenase products
   A. Prostaglandin 2 (PG_2)
   B. Prostaglandin H_2 (PGH_2)
   C. Thromboxane A_2 (TxA_2)
   D. Endoperoxides (vasoconstrictor prostanoids) (F_2 isoprostane)
   E. Arachidonic acid (AA) derivatives

5. Thrombin (T)

6. Nicotine (N)

7. Serotonin (ST) (variable vasoconstriction or vasodilation)

Endothelin-1 (ET-1)[1,4,6,67]
General Points

◆ Most powerful vasoconstrictor known
◆ Produced by activated endothelial cells and VSMC
◆ Binds to receptors on VSMC
◆ Similar to neurotoxins
◆ $T_{1/2}$ 4–7 minutes
◆ Vascular remodeling secondary to Ang-II is mediated by ET-1

Endothelin is Involved in Many Diseases[4]

◆ Hypertension
◆ Pulmonary hypertension
◆ Ischemic cardiomyopathy
◆ Renal insufficiency
◆ Cerebral ischemia
◆ Subarachanoid hemorrhage
◆ Preeclampsia
◆ Congestive heart failure

Three Structurally Distinct Isopeptides[3]

ET-1: Primary vasoconstrictor: ER subtype A
ET-2: Kidney and intestine
ET-3: High concentrations in neuronal cells (especially brain)

Endothelin-Converting Enzyme (ECE)[6]

ECE-1 and ECE-2 catalyze synthesis of ET-1
ECE-1 is a zinc metalloprotease with 40% similarity to neutral endopeptidase

Endothelin Receptors (ET_AR and ET_BR)

ET_AR: On VSMC. Causes Vasocontriction

ET_BR: On endothelium and VSMC

◆ Endothelial ET_BR increases EDHF and PGI_2 and vasodilation

◆ VSMC ET_BR causes vasocontriction

Stimuli for Production[1,3,4,6,67]

Ang-II via AT_1R and other pathways
Catecholamines
Growth factors (TGF-β)
Hypoxia
Insulin
Shear stress and distention of arteries
Thrombin
Endotoxins
Adrenaline
Vasopressin
TGF-β
IL-1B
oxLDL-C
CHF
Cytokines (IL-2 and others)

Inhibitors of Production

NO (via cGMP)
PGI_2 (via cGMP and cAMP)
ANP

Mechanism of Action[4]

Modulates ion channels
Depends on presence of calcium (Ca^{2+})
Promotes Ca^{2+} uptake into cells by two mechanisms:
    A. Through Ca^{2+} channels (role of CCB)
    B. Direct Ca^{2+} mobilization independent of Ca^{2+} channels

Discussion

Endothelin is the most potent vasoconstrictor yet identified. Numerous stimuli cause its production. In hypertensive patients, stimulation of the AT1R (angiotensin-I receptor) increases endothelin production. The ARBs block AT1R and lower endothelin production. In addition, by reducing ROS and O_2^-, the ARBs reduce oxLDL, cytokines, TGF-B, and IL-TB, which contribute to endothelin production as well.

Endothelin: Production Pathway[1,5,6,27]

Requires *de novo* protein synthesis after expression of endothelin gene.

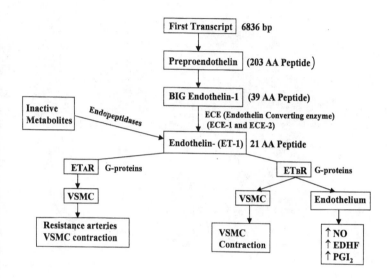

ET$_A$R, endothelin A receptor; ET$_B$R, endothelin B receptor; VSMC, vascular smooth muscle cell; NO, nitric oxide; EDHF, endothelium-dependent hyperpolarizing factor; PGI$_2$, prostacyclin.

Endothelin Pathways[5]

Interaction Between Endothelin-1 and Endothelium-Derived Relaxing Factors

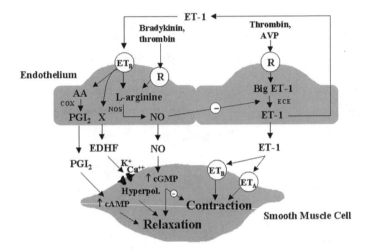

AA, arachidonic acid; cAMP, cyclic AMP; cGMP, cyclic GMP; EDHF, endothelium-derived hyperpolarizing factor; ET, endothelin, endothelin receptor; hyperpol., hyperpolarization; K^+Ca^{2+}, calcium-dependent potassium channel; NO, nitric oxide; NOS, nitric oxide synthase; PGI_2, prostacyclin; R, receptor; X, unknown precursor.

Endothelin (ET-1) Effects[4,6]

♦ Vasoconstriction
♦ VSM proliferation
♦ Secretion of extracellular matrix
♦ Mitogen role, especially in atheroma plaque
♦ Hormone production

Clinical Treatment Considerations[67]

ET-1 is increased in areas of intimal hyperplasia in atherosclerotic human coronary arteries and aorta.

1. ET-1 → mediates collagen type I synthesis (CT-I)
2. Ang-II → mediates collagen type II synthesis (CT-II)
3. CT-I and CT-II account for most of the hyperplasia and restenosis after PCTA
4. ET-1 is an active mitogen in atheroma plaque

Antihypertensive Therapy Effects

CCB: Most effective available ET-1 inhibitors
Reduce vasoconstriction, vascular remodeling, plaque rupture and restenosis after PCTA
ACEI: ↓ Ang-II, ↓ ET-1, ↓ CT-I, ↓ CT-II
ARB: ↓ Ang-II effects, ↓ CT-I, ↓ CT-II, ↓ ET-1
ERA: ↓ ET-1 effects, ↓ CT-I
ECE-I: ↓ ET-1, ↓ CT-I

Discussion

In this study,[67] human coronary arteries and aortas were shown to have increased CT-1 via endothelin and increased CT-II via Ang II, which contribute to intimal hyperplasia, restenosis after PCTA, and plaque formation and rupture.

Therapeutic combinations of ARB, ACEI, and CCB inhibit Ang-II and ET-1 and reduce CT-I and CT-II formation.

Endothelium Vasoconstrictors and Vasodilators: RAAS[104]

Angiotensin I	Angiotensin (1-7)
Angiotensin II	Angiotensin (1-5)
Angiotensin III	Angiotensin (1-9)
Angiotensin IV	Angiotensin (2-7)
Angiotensin (2-10)	Angiotensin (2-9)
Angiotensin (4-8)	Aldosterone

Renin-Angiotensin-Aldosterone System (RAAS)[47,67,68]

General and Major Points

Two RAAS

1. **Classic RAAS**: BP regulation. Circulating ACE 10%
2. **Tissue RAAS**: Regulates vascular and cardiac structure and function (90%)

Angiotensin-converting enzyme (ACE) is an ectoenzyme that faces lumen of vascular system (i.e., protrudes from cell membranes into extracellular space)

ACE is located on:
1. Vascular endothelial cells: lumen and vasa vasorum
2. Media of VSMC

Angiotensin-II (A-II) is potent vasoconstrictor, growth promoter, thrombogenic, pro-oxidant, proinflammatory, atherogenic hormone

Other types of angiotensins exist with variable cardio-vascular effects, both qualitatively and quantitatively

Aldosterone produces similar cardiovascular effects as A-II

Alternate pathways exist for conversion of A-I → A-II other than ACE

Alternate pathways become quantitatively more important under conditions of disease

RAAS Pathway[47,67,68,104]

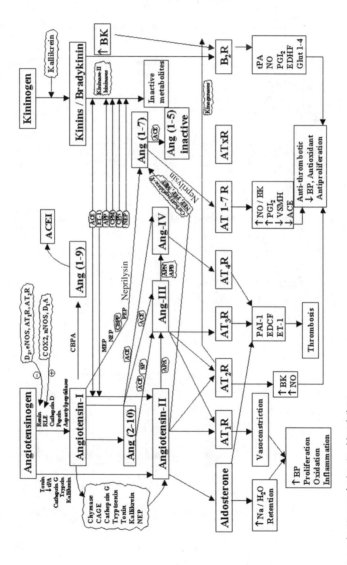

See previous pages for key to abbreviations.

Angiotensin-Converting Enzyme (ACE): Structure and Isoforms[109]

(ACE = Kininase II)

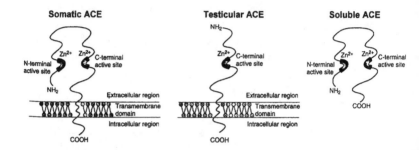

1. **Somatic ACE** (cell-bound ACE, tissue ACE): 170-kDa glycoprotein bilobed ectoenzyme with a homodimeric extracellular region (two homologous domains with two zinc moieties and two active catalytic sites)
2. **Testicular or germinal ACE**: 90-kDa glycoprotein
3. **Plasma ACE** (soluble ACE, circulating ACE): cleaved from somatic ACE

RAAS: ACE Forms[67]

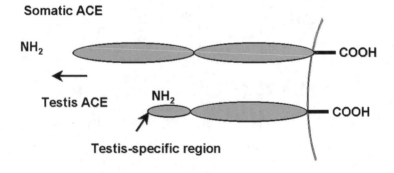

Circulating vs. Tissue ACE[114]

Circulating ACE (endocrine)
- Plasma

Tissue ACE (autocrine/paracrine)
- Vasculature (endothelium)
- CNS
- Adrenal
- Heart
- Kidney
- Reproductive organs
- Lung

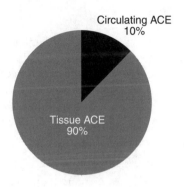

Circulating ACE 10%

Tissue ACE 90%

Endogenous Substrates of ACE and Their Cleavage Sites[109]

Peptide	Sequence
Angiotensin I	H-Asp-Arg-Val-Tyr-Ile-His-Pro-Phe-His-Leu-OH
Bradykinin	H-Arg-Pro-Pro-Gly-Phe-Ser-Pro-Phe-Arg-OH
Des-Arg bradykinin	H-Arg-Pro-Pro-Gly-Phe-Ser-Pro-Phe-OH
β-Neoendorphin	H-Tyr-Gly-Gly-Phe-Leu-Arg-Lys-Tyr-Pro-OH
Dynorphin	H-Tyr-Gly-Gly-Phe-Leu-Arg-Arg-Ile-OH
Enkephalins	
Pentapeptide	H-Tyr-Gly-Gly-Phe-Met-OH
Heptapeptide	H-Tyr-Gly-Gly-Phe-Met-Arg-Phe-OH
Octapeptide	H-Tyr-Gly-Gly-Phe-Met-Arg-Gly-Leu-OH
Chemotactic peptide	N-formyl-Met-Leu-Phe-OH
Neurotensin	pGlu-Leu-Tyr-Glu-Asn-Lys-Pro-Arg-Arg-Pro-Tyr-Ile-Leu-OH
Substance P	H-Arg-Pro-Lys-Pro-Gln-Gln-Phe-Phe-Gly-Leu-Met-NH$_2$
Cholecystokinin-8	H-Asp-Tyr(SO$_3$H)-Met-Gly-Trp-Met-Asp-Phe-NH$_2$
Bombesin	pGlu-Gln-Arg-Leu-Gly-Asn-Gln-Trp-Ala-Val-Gly-His-Leu-Met-NH$_2$
LHRH	pGlu-His-Trp-Ser-Tyr-Gly-Leu-Arg-Pro-Gly-NH$_2$
HSCRP	N-acetyl-Ser-Asp-Lys-Pro-OH

ACE, angiotensin-converting enzyme; LHRH, luteinizing hormone releasing hormone; HSCRP, hematopoietic stem cell regulatory peptide.

Angiotensin-Converting Enzyme (ACE)[67,109]
(Kininase II)

♦ ACE is an ectoenzyme that faces the lumen of vascular system
♦ Membrane bound metalloenzyme with zinc at the active center (zinc peptidase) (metallopeptidase)
♦ Present in huge excess (> Vmax).
  1. A-I → A-II conversion is instantaneous and complete
  2. A-I is equal to or slightly greater than A-II all the time
  3. Increased circulating or tissue (endothelial) ACE may not increase A-II levels

♦ Polypeptide chain with 2 homologous domains each with an independent catalytic site that generate A-I → A-II equally
♦ Four important functional regions
  1. Amino terminus (NH2): signal sequence leads to protein export
  2. Homologous catalytic domain 1
  3. Homologous catalytic domain 2
  4. Carboxyl (COOH) portion is hydrophobic and anchors to cell membrane

♦ C-terminus accounts for 75% total ACE activity and is largely responsible for A-I → A-II conversion
♦ N-terminus accounts for 25% total ACE activity and is responsible for cleaving other peptide substrates
♦ ACE gene is located on chromosome 17q23 region
♦ ACE gene has 26 exons and 25 introns
♦ Insertion-deletion at intron 16 (287-base pair fragment) determines ACE polymorphism with D allele. D allele is associated with:
  1. Increased MI risk
  2. Nephropathy in IDDM
  3. Glomerular disease and renal deterioration
  4. Not to HBP

Distribution of ACE in Human Tissues and Body Fluids[109]

Source	ACE Isoform
Endothelial Cells	Somatic
Arteries	
Veins	
Epithelial Cells	Somatic
Renal proximal tubules	
Gastrointestinal tract	
Submandibular gland	
Choroid plexus	
Epididymis	
Prostate gland	
Cardiovascular System	Somatic
Heart	
Vascular adventitia	
Adrenal cortex	
Brain	Somatic
Basal ganglia	
Posterior pituitary	
Cerebellum	
Reproductive System	
Testis	Testicular
Seminiferous tubules	
Spermatozoa	
Ovary	Somatic
Corpus luteum	
Follicles	
Fibroblasts and Macrophages	Somatic
Body Fluids	Soluble
Plasma	
Seminal fluid	
Urine	
Amniotic fluid	
Cerebrospinal fluid	
Lymph	

ACE, angiotensin-converting enzyme.

Proposed Functions of Tissue ACE[109]

Site	Function
Cardiovascular System (blood vessels, heart)	Regulation of regional blood flow
	Modulation of local sympathetic activity
	Stimulation of hyperplasia and hypertrophy
	Direct action of angiotensin II
	Growth factors (bFGF, PDGF)
	Activation of proto-oncogenes
	Stimulation of nitric oxide and prostacyclin from the endothelium
	Modulation of inotropic and chronotropic activity of the heart
	Inflammatory mediators
Central Nervous System	Processing of neuropeptides
	Maintenance of fluid and electrolyte balance
	Regulation of systemic blood pressure
	Stimulation of drinking behavior
	Modulation of salt appetite
	Modulation of pituitary hormone release
	Modulation of sensory function
	Regulation of effects on learning and memory
Kidney	Regulation of fluid and electrolyte balance
	Regulation of renal blood flow
	Regulation of glomerular filtration
	Control of renin release
Adrenals	Stimulation of aldosterone synthesis and secretion
	Stimulation of catecholamine release
Reproductive Organs	
Testis	Initiation of spermatogenesis
	Regulation of sperm maturation and motility
	Processing of gonadotrophin
Ovary	Regulation of ovulation
	Stimulation of estrogen
Epithelial Cells	Transportation of ions
	Regulation of peptide metabolism
Fibroblasts and Macrophages	Control of inflammation and tissue repair

ACE, angiotensin-converting enzyme; bFGF, basic fibroblast growth factor; PDGF, platelet-derived growth factor.

ACE and ACEI: Clinical-Basic Science Correlations[67]

Extracellular engagement of ACEI to ACE is a function of:
1. Affinity (tissue selectivity, lipophilicity)
2. Tissue blood flow

ACEIs differ in
1. Enzyme binding affinities (tissue selectivity)
2. On and off rates
3. Duration of action

Tissue ACE and conversion of A-I to A-II is an autocrine, paracrine and intracrine function.

ACEIs interact differently with ACE active sides, depending on their structural configurations (ACE and other endogenous peptide degradation)

RAAS and Other Vasoactive Systems

Schematic of the RAAS and interactions with other vasoactive systems.

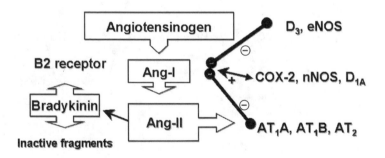

−, Inhibitory effect on renin expression or release; +, stimulatory effect on renin expression or release.

ACE-Independent (Alternate) Pathways for Conversion of AI to AII[47]

Such pathways exist in:

- ♦ Myocardium
- ♦ Coronary arteries
- ♦ Internal mammary arteries
- ♦ Saphenous veins
- ♦ Radial arteries
- ♦ Gastroepiploic arteries

See p. 65.

Metabolism of Angiotensin I (Decapeptide)

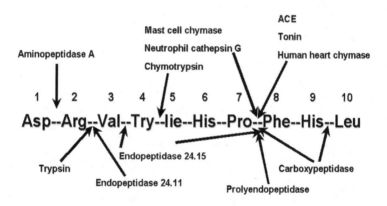

65

Formation of Angiotensins—Alternate Pathways

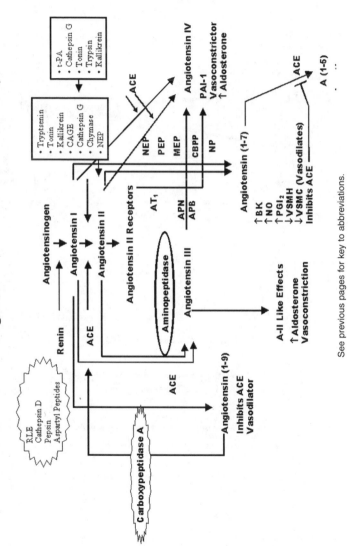

See previous pages for key to abbreviations.

Pathways of Formation of Angiotensins[104]

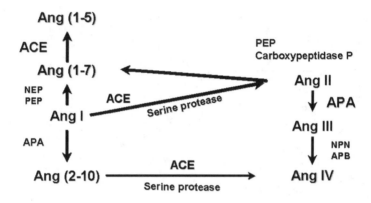

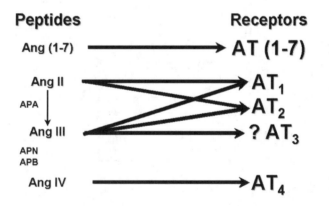

See pages 57 and 69 for vascular effects of the stimulation of the various receptors AT_1R, AT_2R, $ATR(1-7)$, AT_3R, and AT_4R.

Summary
Endothelium Vasoconstrictors;
Endothelin and Others

Endothelin, the most powerful vasoconstrictor known, is produced by activated endothelial cells and VSMC. The vascular effects of Ang-II are mediated by endothelin (ET-1). NO, PGI_2 and ANP are inhibitors of ET-1 production. Antihypertensive drugs such as ARBs, ACEIs, and CCBs, as well as antilipid drugs such as statins, have the ability to reduce ET-1 vascular effects through these and other mechanisms.

The RAAS has become even more complex with over 11 different angiotensins now identified. The classic RAAS is circulating ACE (10% of total ACE) and is primarily concerned with blood pressure regulation. Tissue RAAS (90% of ACE) regulates vascular and cardiac structure and function. Various angiotensin receptors for the different angiotensins have been identified that produce numerous but qualitatively and quantitatively variable cardiovascular effects. The ARBs and ACEs have different effects on the RAAS, on levels of angiotensins, and on angiotensin receptor blockade or stimulation that product favorable vascular biologic results.

c

Chapter 7

The Angiotensins

Nomenclature and Structure of Angiotensin Peptides[104]

Trivial Name	Abbreviation	Systematic Name	Sequence									
			1	2	3	4	5	6	7	8	9	10
Angiotensin I	Ang I, Ang(l-10)	Angiotensin-(1-10) decapeptide	Asp	Arg	Val	Tyr	Ile	His	Pro	Phe	His	Leu
	Ang-(2-10)	Angiotensin-(2-10) nonapeptide		Arg	Val	Tyr	Ile	His	Pro	Phe	His	Leu
Angiotensin II	Ang II, Ang-(1-8)	Angiotensin-(1-8) octapeptide	Asp	Arg	Val	Tyr	Ile	His	Pro	Phe		
Angiotensin III	Ang III, Ang-(2-8)	Angiotensin-(2-8) heptapeptide		Arg	Val	Tyr	Ile	His	Pro	Phe		
Angiotensin IV	Ang IV, Ang-(3-8)	Angiotensin-(3-8) hexapeptide			Val	Tyr	Ile	His	Pro	Phe		
	Ang-(4-8)	Angiotensin-(4-8) pentapeptide				Tyr	Ile	His	Pro	Phe		
	Ang-(1-7)	Angiotensin-(1-7) heptapeptide	Asp	Arg	Val	Tyr	Ile	His	Pro			
	Ang-(1-5)	Angiotensin-(1-5) pentapeptide	Asp	Arg	Val	Tyr	Ile					

Production and Effects of Angiotensin I[104]

Equal vasoconstrictive effect as A-II in:

Saphenous vein
Radial artery
IMA
Coronary artery
Gastroepiploic artery

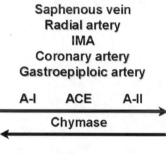

Bidirectional Conversion

Postulated Role of Angiotensin II[104]

Blocking the AT_1R with an ARB results in stimulation of the AT_2R, which has vascular-protective consequences.

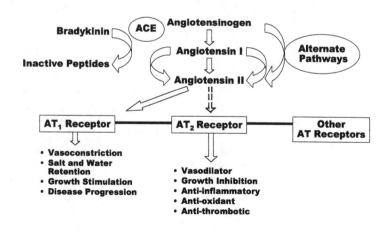

Discussion

Angiotensin II promotes vascular damage in the heart, brain, kidneys, and other organs via vasoconstriction, growth promotion, inflammation, oxidation, and thrombosis.

Angiotensin II (A-II)[4]

A-II causes vasoconstriction, volume overload, increases reactive oxygen species (ROS) and O_2^-, and induces structural and functional changes in cardiac and vascular tissue, such as left ventricular hypertrophy (LVH), vascular remodeling, and renal damage. Adrenergic receptor blockers (ARBs) and angiotensin-converting enzyme inhibitors (ACEIs) can reduce these adverse effects through reduction in blood pressure, ROS, LVH, thrombosis, vascular smooth muscle growth, and glomerular and interstitial sclerosis and fibrosis.

Ang-II

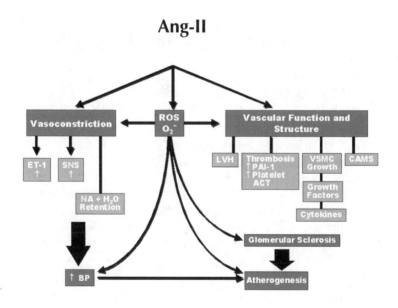

Angiotensin III (A-III)[4,104]

AI $\xrightarrow{\text{ACE}}$ AIII

AII $\xrightarrow{\text{Aminopeptidase}}$ AIII

A-III is qualitatively similar to A-II but quantitatively different:

- It has lower affinity for AT_1R
- Aldosterone secretion: A-II = A-III
- Vasoconstriction: A-III is 10–25% as potent as A-II

Actions of Angiotensin IV (Ang-IV)

Nervous System
- Learning, memory, exploratory behavior
- Inhibition of neurite outgrowth of sympathetic neurons

Cardiovascular System
- Activation of endothelial NOS and cGMP content
- Endothelium-dependent vasodilatation
- Increase in endothelial PAI-I mRNA levels, which increases the risk of thrombosis. The ratio of t-PA to PAI-I determines the relative risk of thrombosis (t-PA/PAI-I ratio).
- Stimulation of hypertrophy/hyperplasia of cardiac fibroblasts
- Antagonism of Ang-II-induced increase in mRNA and protein in chick heart cells
- Dilatation of cerebral vessels

Kidney
- Increase in renal cortical blood flow

Alternate Pathway Enzymes

Chymase[47,68,104]

1. Found in mast cells, endothelial cells, interstitium of heart, and mesenchymal interstitial cells
2. Present in the vasculature of adventitial mast cells
3. Majority of A-II in human myocardium results from chymase generation.

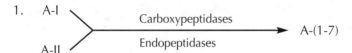

Ang I $\xrightarrow{\text{Chymase}}$ Ang II

4. Chymase is inhibited by serine protease inhibitors
   - Soybean trypsin inhibitor
   - Chymostatin
   - Phenylmethylsulfonyl fluoride
5. Renal A-II formation[104]
   ACE = 2/3
   Non-ACE = 1/3

Other Pathways

1. A-I $\Big\rangle \xrightarrow[\text{Endopeptidases}]{\text{Carboxypeptidases}}$ A-(1-7)
    A-II

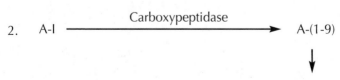

Endopeptidases[47]

- Neutral Endopeptidase (NEP): Endothelium
- Propyl Endopeptidase (PEP): VSMC
- Metalloendopeptidase (MEP): VSMC
- Neprilysin

2. A-I $\xrightarrow{\text{Carboxypeptidase}}$ A-(1-9)

Inhibit ACE
Especially in cardiac myocytes

Alternate Pathway Enzymes[47]
Tonin (T)

◆ Inhibited by alpha macroglobulins

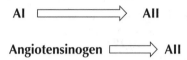

AI ⟹ AII

Angiotensinogen ⟹ AII

Cathepsin G

◆ Mostly found in leukocytes and mast cells

CAGE

◆ CAGE (chymostatin-sensitive Ang-II-generating enzyme)
◆ Derived from mast cells in adventitia of arteries

$$A\text{-}I \xrightarrow[\text{Cathepsin G}]{\text{Tonin}} A\text{-}II$$

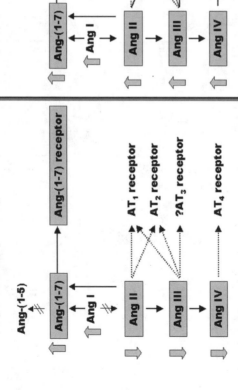

ACE Inhibition [104]

Ang-(1-5)

Ang-(1-7) receptor

Ang-(1-7) ← Ang I

Ang II → Ang III → Ang IV

AT₁ receptor
AT₂ receptor
?AT₃ receptor
AT₄ receptor

Effects of angiotensin-converting enzyme inhibition on angiotensin peptide levels

AT₁ Receptor Antagonism [104]

Ang-(1-7) receptor

Ang-(1-7) ← Ang I

Ang II → Ang III → Ang IV

AT₁ receptor
AT₂ receptor
?AT₃ receptor
AT₄ receptor

Effects of AT₁ receptor antagonism on angiotensin peptide levels

Angiotensin Levels in Humans on ACEI Therapy[104]

Angiotensin peptide levels in cubital venous plasma of normal laboratory personnel (control) and subjects attending a hypertension clinic who were receiving ACEI therapy. *p < 0.05; **p < 0.01.

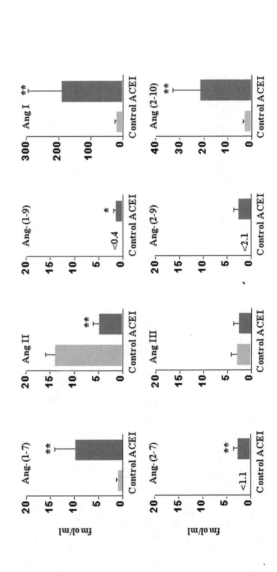

Rationale for Therapy: ACEI + ARB

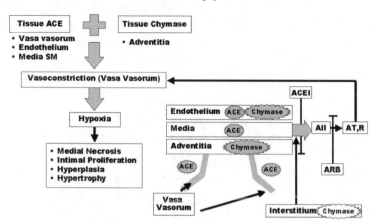

Discussion

Both published (ELITE I, ELITE II, VALHFT) and unpublished studies indicate a role for combination ARB + ACEI in hypertension, congestive heart failure, and renal insufficiency with or without proteinuria. These early beneficial effects of combined therapy require more studies with larger numbers of patients, various drug combinations and doses, and surrogate and hard clinical outcomes.

Rationale for Therapy: ACEI + ARB and ACE, Chymase, Mast Cell[47]

Coronary Arteries: Severity of Disease

1. Early and Intermediate Lesions
ACE primarily in regions of fat-laden macrophages in association with T-lymphocytes.
Mast cells contain ACE and chymase.

2. Severely Diseased Lesions
ACE and A-II localized to endothelial cells lining the microvessels impregnating the plaque
Mast cells: contain ACE + chymase

78

Rationale for Therapy: ACEI + ARB

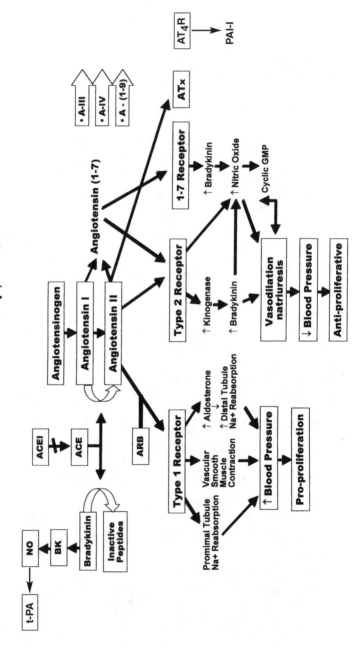

Aldosterone

- ◆ Cardiovascular effects are similar to AII
- ◆ eNOS and NO reduce aldosterone secretion in zona glomerulosa (ZG) adrenal cells
- ◆ NO works via cytochrome P450 enzymes

Cyclo-oxygenase Products:[46]
PG_2, PGH_2, TxA_2, EP, AA, F_2IP

Aging and vascular disease cause:

- ◆ ↑ ROS
- ◆ ↑ O_2^-
- ◆ ↓ NO
- ◆ ↑ PGH_2 (↑ Prostaglandin H synthase (PHHS)

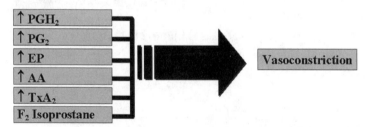

Summary
The Angiotensins

At least 11 different angiotensin peptides have been identified to date, each with specific enzymatic production pathways and cardiovascular and vasomotor effects as shown below:

1. Ang I	Vasoconstrictor	7. Ang-(1-7)	Vasodilator
2. Ang II	Vasoconstrictor	8. Ang-(1-5)	Inactive (?)
3. Ang III	Vasoconstrictor	9. Ang-(1-9)	Vasodilator
4. Ang IV	Vasoconstrictor	10. Ang-(2-7)	Unknown
5. Ang-(2-10)	Vasoconstrictor (?)	11. Ang-(2-9)	Unknown
6. Ang-(4-8)	Unknown		

Chapter 8
Ion Channels and Vascular Tone

Regulation of Vascular Tone[22]

1. VSMC contraction depends on:
   - Calcium influx and intracellular release (storage)
   - Membrane potential: hyperpolarization, depolarization
   - Sensitivity of internal contractile machinery to Ca^{2+}

2. VSMC channels within their plasma membranes
   - K^+ channels (KATP, BKCA, KV, KIR)
   - Ca^{2+} channels (L-type, T-type) (SOC, SAC)
   - Stretch-activated cation channels
   - Chloride (Cl^-) channels (CLCA, CLVR)

3. K^+ channels dominant in VSMC (regulate vascular tone, membrane potential)

4. K_{ATP} response to agonists is blunted in DM

5. BK_{Ca} channel expression increased in VSMC in HBP

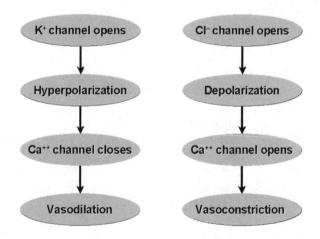

K+ Channels and Vascular Tone[22]

Schematic of a vascular smooth muscle cell (top) and cross-sections through an arteriole (bottom) that shows that opening of K+ channels leads to diffusion of K+ ions out of the cell, membrane hyperpolarization, closure of voltage-gated Ca^{2+} channels, decreased intracellular Ca^{2+}, etc., which leads to vasodilatation. Closure of K+ channels has the opposite effect.

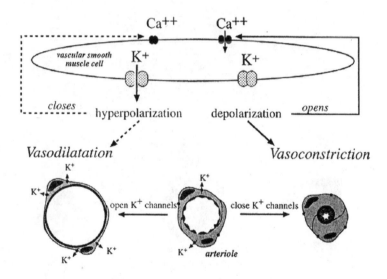

Cl⁻ Channels and Vascular Tone[22]

Schematic of a vascular smooth muscle cell (top) and cross-sections through an arteriole (bottom) that shows that opening of Cl⁻ channels leads to diffusion of Cl⁻ ions out of the cell, membrane depolarization, opening of voltage-gated Ca^{2+} channels, increased intracellular Ca^{2+}, etc., which leads to vasoconstriction. Closure of Cl⁻ channels has the opposite effect.

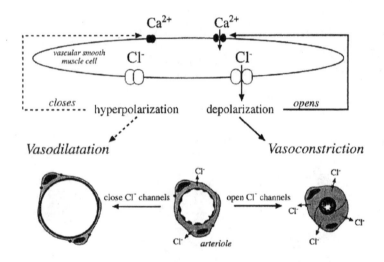

Ca²⁺ Channels[22]

1. **Voltage-gated (VG) Ca2+ channels**
   - L-type (dihydropyridine [DHP]-sensitive)
   - T-type

2. **Store-operated Ca²⁺ channels (SOCC)**

3. **Stretch-activated Ca²⁺ channels (SACC)** (operate even in presence of DHP calcium channel blockers)

Regulation of Ca²⁺ Channels[22]

Agents that increase calcium influx or intracellular release (vasoconstrict):

- Protein kinase C (PKC)
- Inositol 1,4,5-triphosphate (IP_3)
- 20-Hydroxyarachidonic acid (20-HETE)
- Diacylglycerol (DAG)
- Phospholipase C (PLC)
- Adenosine triphosphate (ATP)

Agents that decrease calcium influx or intracellular release (vasodilate):

- Protein kinase A (PKA)
- Protein kinase B (PKB)
- Prostaglandin I_2 (PGI_2)
- Adenosine (cAMP, PKA)
- Carbon monoxide (CO)
- Cyclic adenosine monophosphate (cAMP)
- Cyclic guanosine monophosphate (cGMP)
- Isoproterenol
- Pinacidil
- Nitric oxide (NO)

Ion Channels and Vascular Tone[22]

Schematic of a cross-section through part of a vascular muscle cell. K_{IR}, K_{ATP}, K_V, and BK_{Ca} channels are shown along the top membrane. Also shown are volatge-gated Ca^{2+} channels, two types of Cl^- channels, store-operated calcium channels (SOCC), and stretch-activated calcium channels (SACC). Shown in the membranes of the sarcoplasmic reticulum (SR) are ryanodine receptors (RyR) and inositol 1,4,5-triphosphate (IP_3P). On the bottom membrane, a few of the signals that are known to modulate the function of the ion channels are depicted.

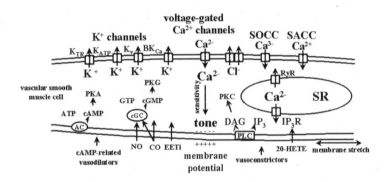

AC, adenylate cyclase; PKA, cAMP-dependent protein kinase; cGS, soluble guanylate cyclase; PKG, cGMP-dependent protein kinase; EETs, epoxyeicotetraenoic acid (epoxides of arachidonic acid); PLC, phospholipase C; DAG, diacylglycerol; PKC, protein kinase C; 20-HETE, 20-hydroxyarachidonic acid.

Summary
Ion Channels and Vascular Tone[22]

Ion channels play a central role in the regulation of vascular tone. Ca^{2+} influx through voltage-gated (VG) calcium channels, store-operated calcium channels (SOCC), and stretch-activated calcium channels (SACC) provides a major source of activator Ca^{2+} used by resistance arteries and arterioles. The K^+ and Cl^- channels and the Ca^{2+} channels all are involved in the determination of the membrane potential of these cells. In turn, membrane potential, with intracellular Ca^{2+}, regulates and modulates Ca^{2+} influx and Ca^{2+} release and Ca^{2+} sensitivity of the contractile machinery. Functions of many of these channels are modulated by the signals and signaling pathways. Thus, ion channels are involved to an important degree in the generation of vascular tone and in neural, humoral, and regulation of this critical variable.

Chapter 9

Endothelial Dysfunction

Definition[105]

The term endothelial dysfunction was proposed to describe the potential for vascular endothelium to undergo phenotypic modulation to a nonadaptive state, characterized by the loss or dysregulation of critical homeostatic mechanisms normally operative in healthy endothelial cells.

◆ Source of biologic response modifiers
1. Endothelial cell (EC)
2. Vascular smooth muscle cell (VSMC)
3. Emigrated leukocytes (EML)

◆ These cells are oxidant stress sensors

Endothelial Dysfunction[1,4,5,6,9,18,105,107]

◆ Characterized by decreased release of relaxing factors (vasodilators) and propensity to secrete contracting factors (vasoconstrictors)
◆ Key and initial earliest event in vascular disease present with only risk factors but no atherosclerosis
◆ Precedes intimal thickening by a decade and clinical atherosclerosis
◆ Correlation with future CV events (MI, PCTA, CABG, sudden death)
◆ Diverse pathophysiologic stimuli are capable of inducing similar nonadaptive changes in endothelial function ("syndrome of endothelial dysfunction"[105,107])
◆ Hypertension (1° and 2°) has reduced endothelial vasodilation (EDV) in both peripheral and coronary arteries[107]

Endothelial Dysfunction[4]

Alterations in viscoelastic properties of arterial wall and reactions to vasoactive stimuli:

1. Thickened subendothelial sheet
2. Increased protein deposition
3. Increased lipid deposition
4. Increased proinflammatory cells
5. Paradoxical vasoconstriction (coronary artery to acetyl-choline), exercise

Grades and Forms of Endothelial Dysfunction

1. Damage of the galphai proteins
2. Decreased release of NO, prostacyclin, EDHF
3. Increase of endoperoxidase discharge
4. Increase of ROS
5. Increase ET-1 production
6. Decrease VSMC sensitivity to NO, prostacyclin, EDHF
7. Activity of kinins holds up in spite of endothelial dysfunc-tion, except in severe arterial lesions

Two Paradigms of Endothelial Activation: Biochemical and Biomechanical[105]

The term **endothelial activation** is used to connote the modulation of endothelial functional phenotype in response to physiologic and pathophysiologic stimuli, which can have both adaptive and non-adaptive consequences. By virtue of its position at the interface between flowing blood and tissues, endothelium is exposed to a vast array of both biochemical and biomechanical stimuli that an induce endothelial activation. The biochemical stimuli (hormones growth factors, cytokines, and bacterial products) can be delivered via the blood and also in an autocrine (acting on the cell of origin) or paracrine (acting on adjacent cells) manner. The biomechanical stimuli consist of wall shear stresses (tractive forces geerated at the luminal endothelial interface by blood flow), pressures (hydrostatic forces that act perpendicular to the endothelial interface), and cyclic strains (circumferential stretching of endothelium and other cells within the vessel wall, as a consequence of pulsatile blood flow).

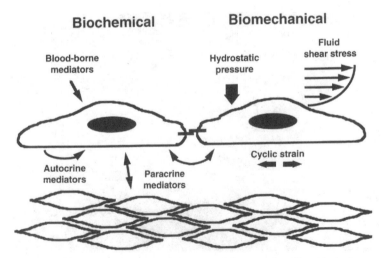

From Gimbrone MA, Topper JN: Biology of the vessel wall: Endothelim. In Chien KR (ed): Molecular Basis of Cardiovascular Disease. Philadelphia, WB Saunders, 1999, p 339, with permission.

Endothelial Dysfunction: Pathophysiologic Stimuli and Consequences[105]

The phenotypic modulation of endothelium to a nonadaptive state in response to certain pathophysiologic stimuli is termed endothelal dysfunction. These biochemical and biophysical stimuli are capable of dysregulating key homeostatic balances that underlie the vital functions of vascular endothelium. The pathophysiologic consequences of endothelial dysfunction include many of the hallmarks of chronic vascular disease, such as altered permeability to plasma macromolecules (e.g., low-density lipoprotein), thrombosis, inflammation, abnormal vasoreactivity, and intimal hyperplasia (smooth muscle migration and proliferation) and fibrosis (extracellular matrix production).

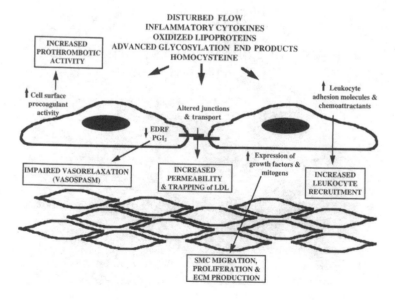

From Gimbrone MA, Topper JN: Biology of the vessel wall: Endothelim. In Chien KR (ed): Molecular Basis of Cardiovascular Disease. Philadelphia, WB Saunders, 1999, p 334, with permission.

Endothelial Dysfunction

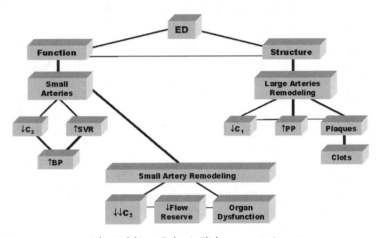

Adapted from Cohn J: Slide presentation at
International Society of Hypertension, August 2000.

Causes and Consequences of Endothelial Dysfunction

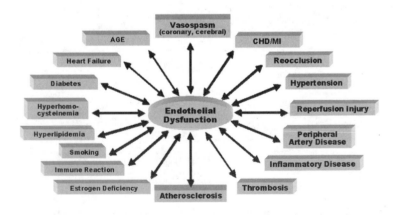

Adapted from Rubanyi GM: The role of endothelium in cardiovascular
homeostasis and diseases. J Cardiovasc Pharmacol 1993; 22(Suppl 4):S1–S4.

Atherosclerosis Timeline

- Atherosclerosis occurs slowly over decades beginning with a mild form of endothelial injury that alters function. Foam cells are the earliest sign of endothelial dysfunction (macrophages that contain oxidized LDL-C).

- Foam cells infiltrate the vessel, forming fatty streaks, then to an intermediate lesion with small pools of extracellular lipid within the smooth muscle layers, disrupting the intimal lining.

- Progression to an advanced atheroma occurs when the accumulated lipid, cells, and other components of the plaque disrupt the artery wall.

- The fibrous plaque is prone to rupture.

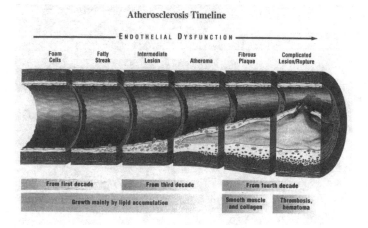

From Pepine CJ: The effects of angiotensin-converting enzyme inhibition on endothelial dysfunction: potential role in myocardial ischemia. Am J Cardiol 1998; 82(10A):23S–27S, with permission.

Discussion

Angiotensin II (Ang-II) promotes atherogenesis through numerous mechanisms. Importantly, LDL-C cannot be oxidized in the absence of Ang-II.

Unifying Model: Endothelial Dysfunction to CVD

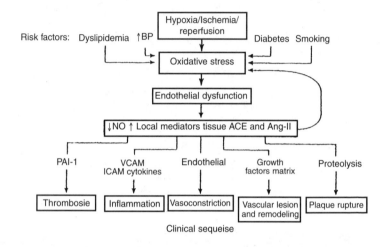

Figure based on data from Gibbons GH, Dzau VJ, N Engl J Med. 1994:330:1431-1438.

Hypertension, dyslipidemia, heart disease, diabetes, and smoking can cause physiologic and structural changes that can lead to atherosclerosis.

Oxidative metabolism in the endothelium causes an increase in the level of oxidative stress. Endothelial cells decrease production of some compounds and increase production of others. NO production is decreased, facilitating vasoconstriction and plaque and thrombosis formation.

Summary
Endothelial Dysfunction

Endothelial activation and subsequent dysfunction constitute a phenotypic modulation of the vascular endothelium to a nonadaptive state characterized by the loss or dysregulation of critical homeostatic mechanisms that normally operate in healthy endothelial cells. Endothelial cells are oxidant stress sensors that react to a host of biochemical and biomechanical mediators, resulting in a myriad of pathophysiological consequences that promote vascular disease, atherosclerosis, and target organ damage by altering vascular function and structure.

Endothelial dysfunction is the key, initial, and earliest event in vascular disease present with only risk factors but no atherosclerosis. It predicts future cardiovascular events but precedes intimal thickening and atherosclerosis by years to decades.

Chapter 10

Atherosclerosis

Atherosclerosis and Inflammation: Endothelial Dysfunction[29]

◆ Atherosclerosis (AS) and inflammation share similar mechanism during the early phases which involve increased interactions between vascular endothelium and circulating leukocytes

◆ Membrane phospholipids are major modulators of cell responsiveness to cytokines

◆ Primary AS site at arterial bifurcations, branch points, convex side with low or oscillatory shear stress favors passive transport of blood components into the vessel wall

◆ Fatty streak is earliest stage of plaque development and is reversible. It is present in 50% of children age 10–14 years on autopsy.

The Inflammatory Response[40,106]

Leukocyte recruitment to the endothelium is mediated by the interaction of adhesion molecule receptors expressed on the surface of endothelial cells with counterreceptors expressed on immune cells.

Leukocyte classes involved in atherogenesis include:

1. **Mononuclear cells**
   Mononuclear phagocytes
   Macrophages
   Monocytes

2. **Lymphocytes**
   T-cells (CD4, CD8)
   Plasma cells
   B-cells

3. **Polymorphonuclear (PMN) cells**
   Granulocytes
   Eosinophils

Endothelial Dysfunction and Atherosclerosis[3,29,35,36]

Atherosclerosis involves endothelial dysfunction and/or damage or death with necrosis or apoptosis. It requires endothelial activation. Endothelial cells undergo morphologic and functional alterations when activated, producing various proteins and immunologic surface markers that augment adhesion and migration reactions of leukocytes that start the atherosclerotic process. Cytokines, other biohumoral mediators, and flow sensors and receptors coupled to nuclear events and signal transduction pathways produce these changes.

Two Paradigms of Endothelial Activation: Biohumoral and Biomechanical[3]

Vascular endothelium is located at the critical interface between blood and tissues, in a key position to respond to stimuli of both kinds. On the one hand, biochemical mediators (such as cytokines) may arrive at endothelial cells from circulating blood or from abluminal sites (from neighboring cells such as leukocytes, pericytes, smooth muscle cells), and may act in an autocrine or paracrine manner. On the other hand, endothelial cells may be subjected to biomechanical forces, which are generated from the pulsatile blood flow, and which comprise the shear stress of circulating blood, hydrostatic pressure and cyclic strains. Both types of stimuli may lead to activation or repression of specific genes.

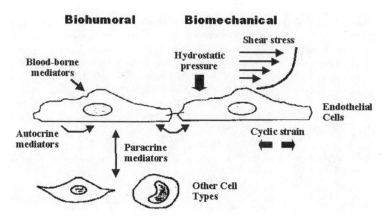

Endothelial–Leukocyte Interaction

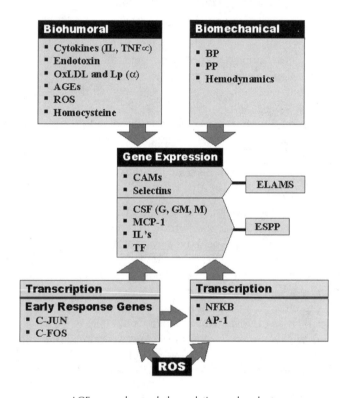

AGE=	advanced glycosylation endproducts
IL=	interleukins
TNF=	tissue necrosis factor
AP-1=	activator protein 1
ELAMS=	endothelial cell leukocyte adhesion molecules
ESPP=	endothelial cell soluble protein products
NFKB=	nuclear factor kappa B
OXLDL=	oxidized low-density lipoprotein
Lp(a)=	lipoprotein (a)
ROS=	radical oxygen species
BP=	blood pressure
PP=	pulse pressure
CAM=	cell adhesion molecules
CSF=	colony-stimulating factor
MCP=	monocyte chemoattractant protein

Cytokines

Definition[3,35,103,106]

Small proteins with multiple biologic activities, active at low (pico-molar) concentrations, produced by immunologically active cells in response to external stimuli (infection, inflammation, endo-exotoxin) that contribute to immune responses, shock inflammation, endothelial cell activation and atherosclerosis, CHD, MI, CHF, and endothelial dysfunction. Cytokines mediate inflammation and immunity.

Mechanism and Location[3,35,103]

◆ Arrive at endothelial cells from
  1. Circulating blood
  2. Endothelium
  3. Abluminal sites (leukocytes, pericytes, VSMCs, macrophages, fibroblasts)
◆ Act in autocrine or paracrine manner

Classification[3,35,63]

◆ **Proinflammatory Cytokines**
  1. Interleukin 1 (IL-1)
  2. Interleukin 6 (IL-6)
  3. Interleukin 8 (IL-8)
  4. Tumor necrosis factor-alpha (TNF-α)

◆ **Colony-Stimulating Factors**
  1. Granulocyte colony-stimulating factor (G-CSF)
  2. Monocyte colony-stimulating factor (M-CSF)
  3. Granulocyte-monocyte colony-stimulating factor (GM-CSF)

◆ **Chemotactic Factors (Chemoattractants)**
  1. Monocyte chemoattractant protein-1 (MCP-1)
  2. Macrophage inhibitory protein-1B (MIP-1B)
  3. Platelet-activating factor (PAF)
  4. Leukotriene-B4 (L-B4)
  5. Complement components
  6. N-formyl peptides
  7. GRO-α

Cell Adhesion Molecules (CAMs)[38,39,41]

The molecular interactions responsible for cellular adhesion (either cell–cell or cell–extracellular matrix) are well orchestrated and under sophisticated control of cell adhesion molecules (CAMs). These molecules include cadherins, integrins, selectins, and the immunoglobulin superfamily. They serve a broad range of biologic processes including platelet aggregation, hemostasis, leukocyte adhesion and extravasation, immune response, inflammation, and maintenance of endothelial and vascular integrity. Disease states may result from loss of adhesion interaction or stimulation of excessive adhesion. High levels of CAMs correlate with vascular diseases and conditions such as atherosclerosis (vascular cell adhesion molecule-1, intracellular adhesion molecule-1), diabetes mellitus, hyperlipidemia, hypertension, coronary heart disease, percutaneous transluminal angioplasty/restenosis.

Multiple Protein Families of Endothelial Surface CAMs[3,28,38]

- ◆ **Selectins** (slowing and rolling of leukocyte on endothelium)
  1. P-selectin (platelet/endothelium selectin)
  2. E-selectin (endothelial selectin)
  3. L-selectin (leukocyte selectin)
  4. CD-34 (Cluster of differentiation 34)

- ◆ **Immunoglobulin superfamily** (adhesion, immune response, inflammation, atherosclerosis)
  1. ICAM-1 to ICAM-5 (Intracellular CAMs)
  2. VCAMs (vascular CAMs)
  3. MADCAM-1 (Mucosal-adhesion CAM)
  4. PECAM-1 (Platelet-endothelial CAM)

- ◆ **Cadherins** (epithelial integrity and correct architecture)
  1. N, P, R, B, and E cadherins
  2. Desmogleins 1 and 3
  3. Desmocollins

- ◆ **Integrins** (external cell membrane to internal signal proteins)
  1. β_1 (leukocyte–ECM) VLA
  2. β_2 (leukocyte–ICAM)
  3. β_3 (Platelets)
  4. β_4–β_8
  5. Subunits attached to all beta subunits (> 20 types)

Selected Endothelial-Leukocyte Adhesion Molecules, Endothelial Chemoattractants and Their Cognate Ligands Implicated in Atherosclerosis[3]

Gene Family		CD Nomenclature	Cell/Tissue Expression	Cognate Ligand
Surface-associated				
Integrins	β2	CD11a/CD18 (LFA-1)	Leukocytes (monocyte, lymphocyte)	ICAM-1, -2 and -3
		CD11b/CD18 (Mac-1)	Leucocytes (monocyte)	
		CD11c/CD18	Leucocytes (monocyte)	
	β1	α4β1 (VLA-4)	Leucocytes (monocyte, lymphocyte)	
Selectins		L-selectin (CD62L)	Leukocytes	Sialyl Lewis and Lewis
		E-selectin (ELAM-1, CD62E)	Endothelium	Sialyl Lewis and Lewis
		P-selectin (CD62P, PADGEM)	Endothelium platelets	Sialyl Lewis and Lewis
Immunoglobulins		ICAM-1	Endothelium and certain leukocyte cell lines	LFA-1 and Mac-1
		ICAM-2	Endothelium, platelets	LFA-1 and Mac-1
		ICAM-3	Leucocytes	
		VCAM-1	Endothelium, smooth muscle	VLA4
		PECAM-1 (CD31)	Endothelium, platelets, leukocytes	
Mucin-like		PSGL-1	Leukocytes	P-selectin
Secreted				
Cylokine		IL-1	Monocytes, smooth muscle	IL-1 receptor
		TNF	Monocytes, smooth muscle	TNF receptor
		MCP-1	Endothelium smooth muscle	MCP-1 receptor
		M-CSF	Endothelium smooth muscle	M-CSF receptor
Lipid		PAF	Endothelium, leukocytes	PAF receptor

ELAM, endothelial leukocyte adhesion molecule; ICAM, intracellular adhesion molecule; IL, interleukin; LFA, leukocyte function-associated antigen; MCP, monocyte chemoattractant protein; M-CSF, macrophase colony-stimulating factor; VCAM, vascular cell adhesion molecule; PAF, platelet-activating factor; PECAM, platelet-endothelial cell adhesion molecule; TNF, tumor necrosis factor; VLA, very late activation antigen.

Integrins

The figure below shows the organization of the integrin family of proteins. The integrins can be subdivided into groups based on the beta subunits. Most of the beta subunits are shared by more than one alpha subunit. This remains an evolving family of proteins.

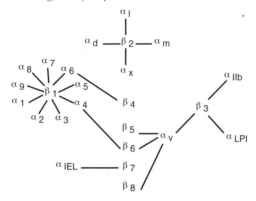

Integrin Taxonomy and Ligands[41]

Integrin Subfamilies	Ligands
β_1 sufamily (VLA)	
$\alpha_1\beta_1$ (VLA-1, CD49a)	Laminin, collagen
$\alpha_2\beta_1$ (VLA-2, GPIa, CD49b)	Collagen, laminin
$\alpha_3\beta_1$ (VLA-3, CD49c)	Fibronectin, laminin, collagen
$\alpha_4\beta_1$ (VLA-4, CD49d)	Fibronectin, VCAM-1
$\alpha_5\beta_1$ (VLA-5, GPIc, CD49e)	Fibronectin
$\alpha_6\beta_1$ (VLA-6, GPIc', CD49f)	Laminin
β_2 sufamily (leukocyte integrins)	
$\alpha_L\beta_2$ (LFA-1, CD11a)	ICAM-1, ICAM-2
$\alpha_M\beta_2$ (Mac-1, CD11b)	ICAm-1, iC3b, fibrinogen, Factor X
$\alpha_x\beta_2$ (p150, CD11c)	Fibrinogen, iC3b,
$\alpha_D\beta_2$	ICAM-3
β_3 sufamily (cytoadhesins)	
$\alpha_{IIb}\beta_3$ (GP IIb, CD41)	Fibrinogen, fibronectin, vitronectin, von Willebrand factor
$\alpha_v\beta_3$ (vitronectin receptor, CD51)	Fibrinogen, fibronectin, vitronectin, von Willebrand factor, thrombospondin, osteopontin

GP, glycoprotein; ICAM, intracellular adhesion molecule; LFA, leukocyte function association; VCAM, vascular cell adhesion molecule; VLA, very late activation.

Integrin Subunits, Ligands, and Cellular Distribution[41]

Subunit		Ligands	Cellular Distribution	
			Nonleukocyte	Leukocyte
β_1	α_1	CO, laminin	F, BM	actB, actT
	α_2	CO, laminin	P, F, EN, EP	actT
	α_3	Fibronectin, laminin, CO	EP, F	
	α_4	Fibronectin, VCAM-1	NC, F	B, T, M, LGL
	α_5	Fibronectin	F, EP, EN, P	Th, T
	α_6	Laminin	P	T
	α_7	Laminin	MYO, EP	
	α_8	OP, vitronectin, fibronectin	EP, NC	
	α_v	Fibronectin, OP, vitronectin	F	
β_2	α_L	ICAM-1, ICAM-2, ICAM-3		B, T, M, G
	α_M	C3b, fibrinogen, factor X, ICAM-1		M, G
	α_X	C3b, fibrinogen		M, G
β_3	α_{IIb}	Fibronectin, fibrinogen, vWF, vitronectin, thrombospondin	P	
	α_v	OP,CO	EN	
β_4	α_6	Laminin	C	
β_5	α_v	Fibronectin, vitronectin	C, F, EP	
β_6	α_v	Fibronectin	C, EP	
β_7	α_4	Fibronectin		IEL
	α_E	E cadherin		IEL
β_8	α_v	Fibronectin, VCAM-1, laminin		

actB, activated B cells; actT, activated T cells; B, B cells; BM, basement membranes; c, carcinoma cells; CO, collagens; EN, endothelium; EP, epithelium; F, fibroblasts; G, granulocytes; IEL, intraepithelial lymphocytes; LGL, large granular lymphocytes; M, monocytes; MYO, myocytes; NC, neural crest-derived cells; OP, osteopontin; P, platelets; T, T cells; Th, thymocytes.

Signaling Mechanisms[38,39]

Inside-Out and Outside-In Signals

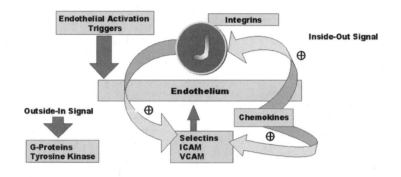

VCAM-1/VLA-4 integrin interaction is specific for early atherosclerosis and mononuclear recruitment.

Integrin Signaling Mechanisms[41]

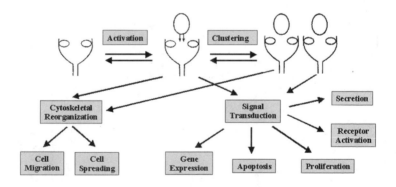

Phases of Leukocyte–Endothelium Interactions[29]

1. Rolling: initial transient adhesion
2. Activation
3. Adhesion, arrest, and spreading
4. Diapedesis: transendothelial migration

ATHERO-ELAMs (endothelium-leukocyte adhesion molecules)

Monocyte recruitment and arterial intima is specific to atherosclerosis. Specific expression of ELAMS is key. V-CAM-1 expressed early and is the only molecule selective for monocytes.

ESPPs (endothelial soluble proatherogenic products)

Endothelium–Leukocyte (Monocyte) Binding[29]

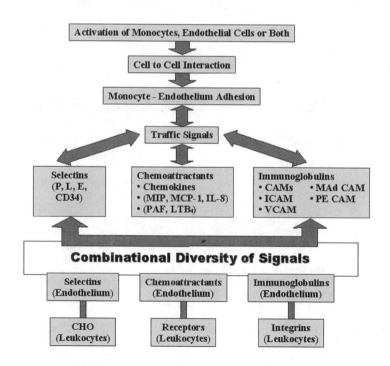

Sequential Steps of Leukocyte Adhesion[41]

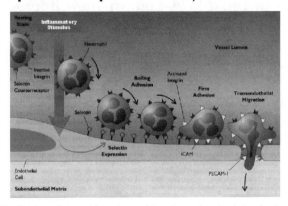

Cell-to-cell adhesions that enable a neutrophil to leave the circulation begin with both the neutrophil and the vascular endothelium in a resting, noninteractive state. Activated by an inflammatory stimulus, the endothelium expresses selectins, whose binding to their receptors on neutrophils initiates a rolling adhesion of neutrophils to the vessel's luminal wall. The neutrophils activate their integrins, which bind to endothelial ICAMs, permitting a firmer, stationary adhesion. Transepithelial migration may be guided by further adhesive interactions, perhaps involving molecules such as PECAM-I, which endothelial cells express at intercellular junctions.

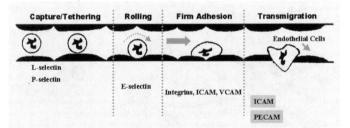

The four-step model of leukocyte adhesion and transmigration across an endothelial monolayer under dynamic flow conditions at sites of inflammation. **Leukocyte tethering and rolling** (steps 1 and 2) are mediated primarily by selectin–carbohydrate interactions, although knock-out murine models suggest that immunoglobulin family members may participate in this step. Also, $\alpha_4\beta_1$ integrins, not expressed by resting neutrophils, are also capable of initiating primary lymphocyte adhesion to endothelial cells through binding to VCAM-1. **Firm adhesion** (step 3) follows if leukocytes encounter activating signals while rolling along the endothelium. Activation-dependent attachment of β_2 integrins (Mac-1, LFA-1) on neutrophils to endothelial ICAM-1 supports this firm or secondary cell adhesion to the vessel wall. Monocytes and lymphocytes may use the $\alpha_4\beta_1$/VCAM-1 pathway in this step. **Transmigration** (step 4) may occur if a favorable chemotactic gradient exists across the monolayer. Platelet/endothelial cell adhesion molecule 1 (PECAM-1) expressed at endothelial cell junctions appears to be required for transmigration by binding homophilically to PECAM-1 expressed on leukocytes. Also, antibodies against β_2/ICAM-1 pathway that block firm adhesion exert a similar effect on neutrophil transendothelial migration.

Endothelial Activation: Adhesive Interactions During Leukocyte (Monocyte) Emigration[29]

Series of events as identified by intravital microscopic studies under flow. The adhesive interactions involved in leukocyte emigration involve several distinct phases: (1) initial transient adhesion (rolling), (2) activation, (3) firm adhesion (arrest and spreading), and (4) transendothelial migration (diapedesis).

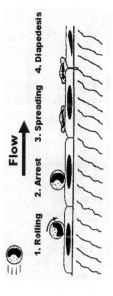

Flow

1. Rolling 2. Arrest 3. Spreading 4. Diapedesis

Molecules Involved

	Rolling	Activation	Firm Adhesion	Transendothelial Migration
Leukocyte	sLex and other sialylated, fucosylated structures	Cytokine, chemokine, and chemoattractant receptors	β_1, β_2, and β_3 integrins	PECAM-1, β_1 and β_2 integrins
	L-selectin			
Endothelial	P-selectin	Chemokines (e.g., IL-8,	ICAM-1, ICAM-2,	PECAM-1
	L-selectin ligand	MCP-1, MIP-1β)	VCAM-1, MAdCAM-1	ICAM-1
	E-selectin	PAF		VCAM-1
	CD34	PECAM-1		
	MAdCAM-1	E-selectin		

Recent in vitro and in vivo studies indicate that rolling is mediated by multiple low-affinity interactions between selectin receptors and their cognate carbohydrate ligands. Firm adhesion and diapedesis are largely dependent on integrin and immunoglobulin-like proteins. CD34, cluster of differentiation 34; PECAM, platelet-endothelial cell adhesion molecule; ICAM, intercellular adhesion molecule; IL, interleukin; MAdCAM, mucosal adhesion cell adhesion molecule 1; MCP, monocyte chemoattractant protein; MIP, macrophage inhibitory protein; PAF, platelet activity factor; sLex, sialyl Lewis; VCAM, vascular cell adhesion molecule.

VCAM-1/Oxidation/NF-κB and Atherosclerosis[40]

Localized Endothelial Expression of VCAM-1 and Selective Exclusive Recruitment of Mononuclear Leukocytes to Vascular Lesions in Early Atherosclerosis

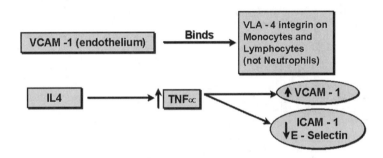

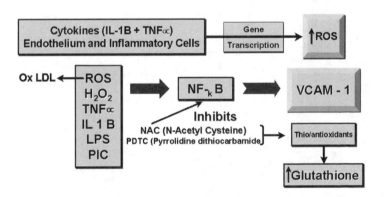

Antioxidants may function by blocking specific, intracellular, redox-sensitive signal transduction pathways in atherogenesis.

See previous pages for key to abbreviations.

Hypertension, Hyperlipidemia, and Diabetes Mellitus—Interrelationships [40]

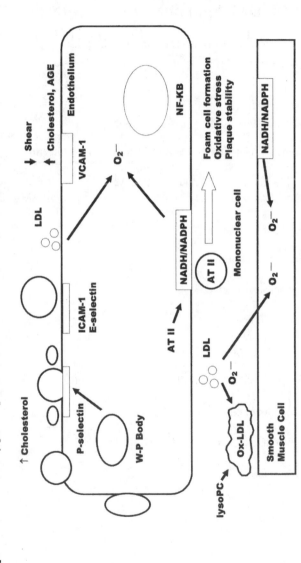

O_2^- is stimulated by oxLDL, A-II, AGEs, and hypertension. O_2^- activates NF-kB, which produces CAMs and cytokines.

Endothelial Injury and Inflammatory Responses in Atherogenesis, Red-OX, HLP, HBP, DM, Smoking , Aging, Infections[41]

Endothelal Dysfunction or Injury

CAMs	Growth Factors	CAMs
↓	↓	↓
Leukocyte adhesion (monocytes, T-cells)	VSMC proliferation	Selectins
↓	↓	Immunoglobulin SF
Subendothelial migration	VSMC migration from media into intima: Intimal VSM proliferation mitogens	Integrins
↓		VCAM-1–VLA4
Foam cells (oxLDL) (lipid-laden macrophage)		ICAMs
↓		VCAM-1–LFA-4
Growth factors		
↓		
Neointimal proliferation		

Intimal expansion (foam cells) → Fatty streak

↓

Endothelial thinning

↓

Endothelial retraction/dysfunction

↓

Exposure of foam cells to blood

↓

Macrophage foam cell–platelet interaction

↓

Fibroproliferative lesion

↓

Mature AS lesion

↓

Plaque with fibrous cap

↓

Plaque rupture

↓

Thrombosis

A-II AT$_1$ Receptor Blockade in Early Atherogenesis

Strawn WB, Ferrario CM, et al Circulation. 2000;101:1586-93

A-II and Atherosclerosis

◆ A-II influences endothelial function,[1,2] monocyte activation and binding to endothelial cells.[3]

◆ A-II influences vascular SMC proliferation and migration,[4] and oxidation of LDL.[5]

1. Ferrario CM et al Cardiovasc Risk Factors. 1996;6:299-310
2. Clozel M et al Hypertension. 1991;18:132-41
3. Kim JA et al Biochem Biophys Res Commun. 1996;226:862-8
4. Kubo A et al J Cardiovasc Pharmacol. 1996;27:58-63
5. Yanagitani Y et al Hypertension. 1999;33(ptII):II-335-II-339

◆ ACE mRNA concentrates in human atherosclerotic plaque in the shoulder regions.[1]

◆ Macrophages in atherosclerotic lesions contain A-II.[2]

◆ A-II induced lipid peroxidation entraps LDL and contributes to foam cell formation.[3]

◆ Atherogenesis is associated with up-regulation of AT$_1$ receptors.

1. Fukura et al Hypertension 2000
2. Potter DD et al Circulation. 1998;98:800-7
3. Keidar S et al Arterioscler Thromb Vasc Biol 1996;16:97-105
4. Yang BC et al Arterioscler Thromb Vasc Biol. 1998;18:1433-1439

◆ Losartan, an AT$_1$ receptor blocker, inhibits LDL oxidation and attenuates atherosclerosis
independent of lowering blood pressure in apolipoprotein E deficient mice.[1]

◆ Losartan reduced monocyte activation and adherence to endothelium independently of blood pressure in (mRen-2)27 transgenic hypertensive rats. [2-4]

1. Hayek T et al Cardiovasc Res. 1999 Dec;44(3):579-87
2. Strawn WB et al AM J Hypertens 1997;101(1):51-57

◆ Hypercholesterolemia-induced atherosclerosis in cynomolgus monkeys bears similarities to human disease[1] and is inhibited by ACE inhibitors.[2]

1. Masuda J et al Arteriosclerosis. 1990;10:164-7
2. Song K et al Arteriosclerosis. 1998;138:171-82

Adult Cynomolgus Monkeys
(Macaca fasciliaris)

Purpose:
To more directly evaluate the role of Ang II in atherogenesis and whether AT1 receptor blockage retards atherogenesis by measuring fatty-streak formation, lipoprotein atherogenicity, the activation status of circulating monocytes and platelets, and the levels of circulating adhesion molecules

1. Strawn WB, Ferrario CM, et al Circulation. 2000;101:1586-93

A-II AT$_1$ Antagonist in Experimental Atherosclerosis in Nonhuman Primates

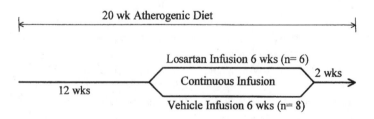

1. Strawn WB, Ferrario CM, et al Circulation. 2000;101:1586-93

A-II Antagonist in Experimental Atherosclerosis in Nonhuman Primates

◆ Losartan infusion (180 mg/day) produced blood levels comparable to 100 mg of losartan dosed once daily in humans.
◆ Two-week recovery period was instituted after cessation of the infusion period.
◆ HPCL used to measure losartan, A-II and A-(1-7).
◆ Blood pressure and heart rate were measured.
◆ Lipids, subfractions and particle size (NMR spectrometry) were measured.

Carlos Ferrario, et al AHA Nov 6, 1999

Changes in Plasma Neurohormones

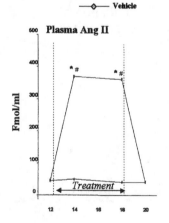
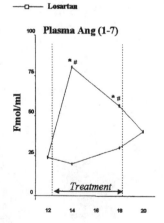

* p< 0.05 comparison within groups vs baseline value
\# p< 0.05 vs vehicle at weeks indicated

Strawn WB, Ferrario CM, et al Circulation. 2000;101:1586-93

◆ Losartan had no effect on DBP, SBP or heart rate.

◆ Losartan raised plasma A-II and A-(1-7).

◆ Losartan reduced plasma cholesterol but not significantly.

◆ No change was observed in lipid subfractions or particle size.

Carlos Ferrario, et al AHA Nov 6, 1999

Effect of Losartan on LDL Oxidation at 6 Weeks' Infusion of Losartan and Vehicle

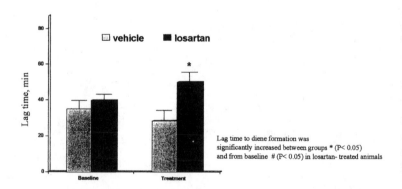

Lag time to diene formation was significantly increased between groups * (P< 0.05) and from baseline # (P< 0.05) in losartan- treated animals

Strawn WB, Ferrario CM, et al Circulation 2000;101:1586-93

Fatty Streak Formation & Composition

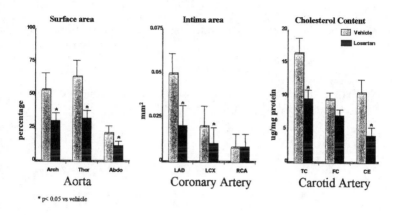

Strawn WB, Ferrario CM, et al Circulation. 2000;101:1586-93

A-II Antagonist on Fatty Streak Formation

◆ Extent of fatty streak formation in the aorta of losartan-treated monkeys was significantly less than in vehicle-treated monkeys (p<0.05).
  ◆ -48% aortic arch
  ◆ -52% thoracic
  ◆ -54% abdominal aorta
◆ Intimal area was less in the LAD and LCx (p<0.05).
◆ Media area was smaller only in the LAD (p<0.05).
◆ Inhibition of fatty-streak formation by losartan was associated with comparatively lower carotid artery content of TC and esterified cholesterol (p<0.05).

Strawn WB, Ferrario CM, et al Circulation. 2000;101:1586-93

Internal Elastic Lamina (IEL)

Vehicle-treated animals

◆ Intimal foam cell accumulation was associated with internal elastic lamina (IEL) disruption and a predominance of α-actin immunopositive cells.

Losartan-treated animals

◆ Reduction of fatty streak macrophage-derived foam cells with no disruption of the IEL.

Strawn WB, Ferrario CM, et al Circulation. 2000;101:1586-93

Losartan on Immune Status and Circulating Markers

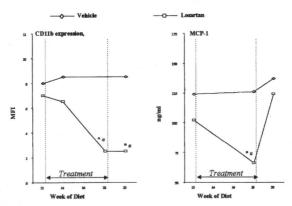

* p< 0.05 comparison within groups vs baseline value
# p< 0.05 vs vehicle at weeks indicated

Strawn WB, Ferrario CM, et al Circulation 2000;101:1586-93

Monocyte Activation and Recruitment

◆ Surface expression of Monocyte Recruitment Factor CD 11b
was significantly reduced by losartan at week 6 of treatment
and at the end of the study ($p < 0.05$).

◆ Adhesion Molecule MCP-1 was reduced by losartan at week 6
of treatment ($p < 0.05$) and returned to pretreatment levels during the recovery phase.

◆ Baseline levels of VCAM-1 and E-Selectin were higher in the
losartan-treated monkeys ($p < 0.05$). Within each treatment
group VCAM-1 and E-Selectin did not significantly differ from
baseline to week 6 of infusion.

◆ Inflammatory marker CRP was unchanged.

Strawn WB, Ferrario CM, et al Circulation. 2000;101:1586-93

Losartan on Immune Status and Circulating Markers

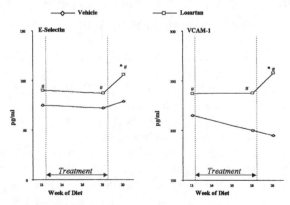

* $p < 0.05$ comparison within groups vs baseline value
# $p < 0.05$ vs vehicle at weeks indicated

Strawn WB, Ferrario CM, et al Circulation 2000;101:1586-93

Representative examples in distribution of sudanophilia within aortas of 4 cholesterol-fed monkeys randomized to either vehicle (a and b) or losartan treatment (c and d)

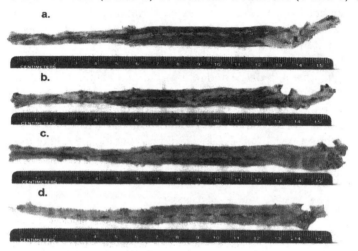

Summary: A-II Antagonist in Experimental Atherosclerosis in Nonhuman Primates

◆ This study demonstrates for the first time in nonhuman primates an antiatherogenic effect of AT1 receptor blockade.

◆ Losartan exerts an inhibitory influence on the early stages of diet-induced atherogenesis through mechanisms that include protection of LDL from oxidation and suppression of vascular monocyte activation and recruitment factors.

◆ Losartan leads to marked reduction in fatty streak production.

◆ Losartan reduces susceptibility of LDL to oxidation.

◆ Losartan retards atherosclerosis development in this model.

◆ The increase in Ang-II and Ang-(1-7) may also contribute to the antiatherogenic actions of losartan, especially when injury-induced vascular smooth muscle cell proliferation is involved,[1] because AT_2 receptor stimulation and Ang-(1-7) administration mediate antiproliferative responses.[2]

1. Strawn WB, Ferrario CM, et al Circulation. 2000;101:1586-93
2. Strawn WB et al Hypertension 1999;33:207-211

Atherosclerosis

- Atherosclerosis is a **disease of the vessel wall**
- It is **NOT** a disease of the lumen
- CHD is an **extraluminal disease**

CHD: Extraluminal Disease: Glagov Principle

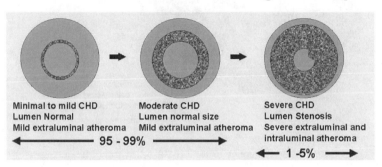

68% of MI: < 50% stenosis; 14% of MI: significant stenosis
MI is the first symptom of CHD in 62% of men and 46% of women
(From lecture by Nissen, S., ISH August 2000.)

Oxiidized LDL-C: A Common Initiating Factor for Cardiac Events

Ox LDL-C is elevated in diseases with increased oxidative stress (dys-lipidemia, hypertension, and diabetes). It induces a chronic inflam-matory reaction in atherosclerotic plaques. Mature plaques contain a large, lipid-filled core with a protective fibrous cap. Mechanical stress and activated macrophages and T-lymphocytes that secrete cytokines weaken the fibrous cap, leading to fragility and rupture and clinical sequelae such as transeint ischemia, unstable ischemic syndromes, myocardial infarction, and death.

Anatomy of Atherosclerotic Plaque

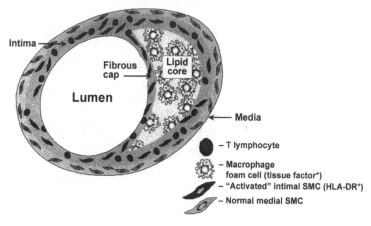

From Libby P: Lancet 1996; 348:S4–S7, with permission.

Characterictics of Plaques Prone to Rupture

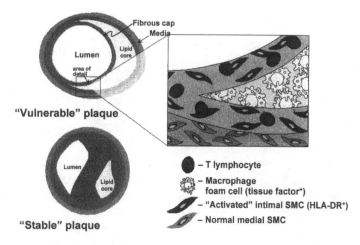

From Libby P: Circulation 1995; 91:2844–2850, with permission.

Angiographically Inapparent Atheroma

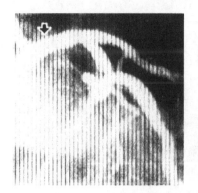
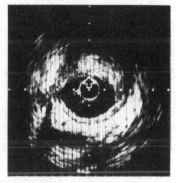

From Topol: Interventional Cardiology Update, 1995, p 14.

Remodeling: Stable and Unstable Lesions: Bidirectional

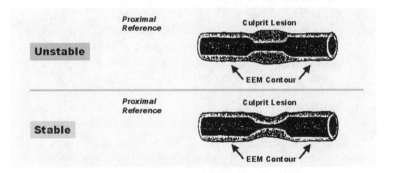

From Nissen H, ISH, August 2000.

Macrophage metalloproteinase 3 (MMP3)

◆ Concentration high in remodeling plaque
◆ Erodes EEM
◆ Causes plaque rupture

120

Prevalence of Atherosclerosis and CHD by Intravascular Ultrasound

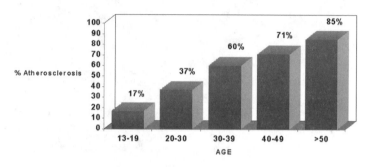

From lecture by Nissen S, ISH, Chicago, August 2000.

Treatment of Endothelial Activation and ED[3]

1. **Decrease intensity or concentration of triggers[4]**
A. Dyslipidemia treatment: ↓ oxLDL, ↓ Lp(a), ↓ TG, ↑ HDL
B. Statins (biologic effects include lipid lowering, improvement of endothelial dysfunction, suppression of inflammatory response in atherosclerotic plaques, increased plaque stability, and inhibition of thrombus formation)
C. DM control: ↓ AGEs
D. ACEI: ↑ NO, ↓ ROS
E. ARB: ↑ NO, ↓ ROS
F. CCB: ↑ NO, ↓ ROS
G. Antioxidants: ↓ oxLDL, ↓ transcription (NF-κB), ↑ NO
H. Homocysteinemia treatment (folate, B_6, folate, B_{12})

2. **Decrease sensitivity of system**
A. OMEGA 3 – PUFA (DHA > EPA) in cell membranes
   ↓ cytokine expression of VCAM-1 50% (NF-κB)
B. Nitric oxide donors stabilize NF-κB
   eNOS + monocytes, macrophages, VSMC (cytokine-iNOS)
C. Estrogens and ERMs
D. CCB
E. Zinc

Treatment of Endothelial Activation and ED[49]

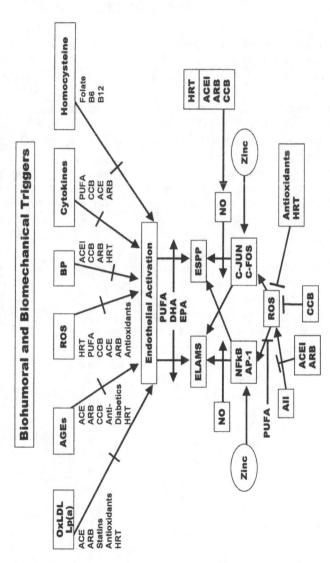

See previous pages for key to abbreviations.
PUFA, polyunsaturated fatty acids; DHA, docosahexaenoic acid; EPA, eicosapentaenoic acid; HRT, hormone replacement therapy.

Summary
Atherosclerosis

Atherosclerosis is an inflammatory disease of the vessel wall (intima and media) that begins at an early age. Endothelial activation and dysfunction initiate the atherosclerotic process following functional and structural changes of the endothelial cell. Various protein molecules and immunologic surface markers augment adhesion and migration of leukocytes, ingestion of oxidized LDL-C by macrophages, foam cell formation, and other events that start the atherosclerotic process.

Cytokines and other biohumoral mediators as well as biomechanical stress (flow sensors and receptors), coupled with signal transduction, nuclear transcription, and specific gene expression, are actively involved in this process.

Treatment of endothelial activation and dysfunction can be directed toward two major areas:

1. Decrease intensity or concentration of triggers
   - A. Hypertension: ARBs, ACEIs, CCBs
   - B. Hyperlipinemia: statins
   - C. Diabetes mellitus: decrease AGEs
   - D. Homocysteine: vitamin B6, B-12, folate
2. Decrease sensitivity of the system
   - A. Omega-3 polyunsaturated fatty acids
   - B. NO bioavailability increased: ARB, ACEI, CCB
   - C. Estrogen and estrogen receptor modulators
   - D. Zinc

Chapter 11

Oxidative Stress and Cardiovascular Disease

Cardiovascular Diseases Related to Increased Oxidative Stress[49,60]

1. Atherosclerosis: oxLDL, Fe in plaque, IC-Ca^{2+}, O$_2^-$, NO
2. Hypertension: ↑O$_2^-$, H$_2$O$_2$, oxLDL, ↓SOD, GTP, A-II, ↓NOS, ↓NO
3. Non-insulin-dependent diabetes mellitus (NIDDM): ↑ROS
4. Acute ischemic syndromes/CHD: ↑O$_2^-$, XO
5. Ischemic reperfusion injury: ↑O$_2^-$, XO
6. Hyperlipidemia: oxLDL
7. CHF: O$_2^-$, ROS

Oxidative Stress and Cardiovascular Disease: Causes and Mechanism[49,60]

Increased oxidative stress (ROS)
1. Increased generation (ROS): ED, AA, catecholamines, etc.
2. Decreased antioxidant reserve
   A. Intracellular (SOD, CAT, GTP)
   B. Extracellular (albumin, TIBC, vitamin C, ceruloplasmin)
   C. Enzymatic and nonenzymatic: vitamin E

Primary and ultimate mechanism of ROS damage
1. Intracellular Ca^{2+} overload via damage of subcellular organelles

Role of Different Extracardiac and Extravascular Systems in the Genesis of Oxidative Stress and Development of Cardiovascular Abnormalities[49]

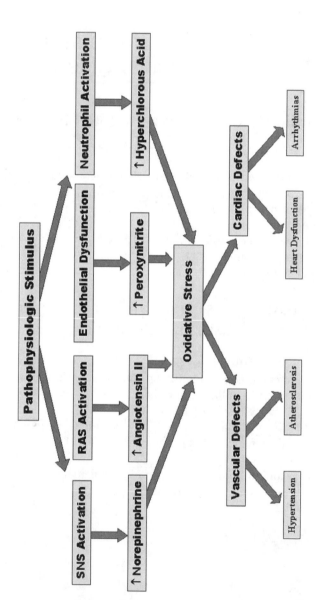

SNS, sympathetic nervous system; RAS, renin-angiotensin system.

Free Radicals, Oxidative Stress, REDOX: Basics[48]

Energy production: Carbonaceous combustion within cells (mitochondria), in favorable thermodynamic reactions allow transfer of electrons or hydrogen atoms to return to molecular O_2 with controlled energy release.

Free radical: Molecule with single unpaired electron
Oxygen is a **diradical—two** electrons are required to form H_2O (substrate–enzyme–O_2 kinetic energy barrier)

REDOX: Reduction-Oxidation Reaction
    Oxidation: loss of electron
    Reduction: gain of electron

Autoxidations:
    Enzymatic: Mitochondrial respiration (ETC leak)
    Nonenzymatic: Stolen electron forms substrate ROS

Free Radical Production: Overview[50]

The active species are the superoxide anion (O_2^-) and hydroxyl free radical (•OH). Hydrogen peroxide (H_2O_2), a relatively weak oxidant, holds a central position in the further metabolism to other ROS or detoxification to water. The fourth ROS, singlet oxygen ($^1O_2$), is not shown.

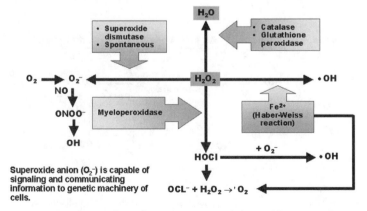

NO, nitric oxide; Fe^{2+}, iron ion; HOCl, hypochlorous acid.

Reactive Oxygen Species (ROS) Production[50]

Many different cellular enzymes catalyze the generation of superoxide anion from molecular oxygen. The membrane-bound NAD(P)H-oxidase is essential for angiotensin II-mediated O_{2-} generation.

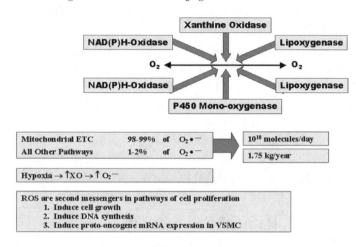

Various Sources of ROS in Health and Disease

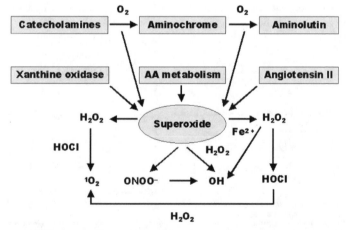

AA, arachidonic acid; HOCl, hypochlorous acid; MPO, myeloperoxidase; ONOO⁻, peroxinitrite.

The Cytotoxic Reactive Oxygen Species and the Natural Defense Mechanisms[49]

Reactive Oxygen Species		Antioxidant Defense Mechanisms	
Free Radicals		*Enzymatic Scavengers*	
$O_2^{\bullet-}$	Superoxide anion radical	SOD	Superoxide dismutase
$OH^{\bullet}$	Hydroxyl radical		$2O_2^{\bullet-} + 2H^+ \rightarrow H_2O_2 + O_2$
$ROO^{\bullet}$	Lipid peroxide (peroxyl)	CAT	Catalase (peroxisomal-bound)
$RO^{\bullet}$	Alkoxyl		$2H_2O_2 \rightarrow O_2 + H_2O$
$RS^{\bullet}$	Thiyl	GTP	Glutathione peroxidase
$NO^{\bullet}$	Nitric oxide		$2GSH + H_2O_2 \rightarrow GSSG + 2H_2O$
$NO_2^{\bullet}$	Nitrogen dioxide		$2GSH + ROOH \rightarrow GSSG + ROH + 2H_2O$
$ONOO^-$	Peroxynitrite		
$CCl_3^{\bullet}$	Trichloromethyl		
		Nonenzymatic scavengers	
		Vitamin A	
		Vitamin C (ascorbic acid)	
		Vitamin E (α-tocopherol)	
Non-radicals		β-carotene	
H_2O_2	Hydrogen peroxide	Cysteine	
HOCl	Hypochlorous acid	Coenzyme Q	
$ONOO^-$	Peroxynitrite	Uric acid	
$^1O_2$	Singlet oxygen	Flavonoids	
		Sulfhydryl group	
		Thioether compounds	

The superscripted bold dot indicates an unpaired electron and the negative charge indicates a gained electron. GSH, reduced glutathione; GSSG, oxidized glutathione; R, lipid chain. Singlet oxygen is an unstable molecule due to the two electrons present in its outer orbit spinning in opposite directions.

Site of Origin of ROS[49,56,58,60]

1. Mitochondrial ETC with impaired reduction of O2
2. Dysfunction endothelium
3. Phagocytic WBC
4. Auto-oxidation of catecholamines
5. Ionizing radiation
6. UV rays
7. Smoking
8. Air pollutants
9. Xanthine oxidase
10. Cyclooxygenase
11. NOS
12. Flavin-containing oxidases
13. Lipooxygenase
14. NAD(P)H oxidase and A-II
15. P450 monooxygenase
16. Growth factors: PDGF
17. Oleic acid and nonesterified FA (NEFA)58
18. Atherosclerotic vessels (XO, NAD(P)H oxidase, oxidases)

ROS Effects on Oxidative Stress and CV Disease[49,60]

1. Lipid peroxidation (PUFA in membrane lipid bilayer)
2. Protein oxidation: induces lipid and CHO auto-oxidation proteolysis
3. Carbohydrate oxidation
4. DNA oxidation and damage
5. Organic molecule oxidation
6. Genetic machinery and gene expression
7. Transcription factors and DNA synthesis

ROS and Subcellular Organelle Defects[49]

Involvement of defects in subcellular organelles due to oxidative stress as a consequence of either increased formation of reactive oxygen species and/or decreased antioxidant reserve.

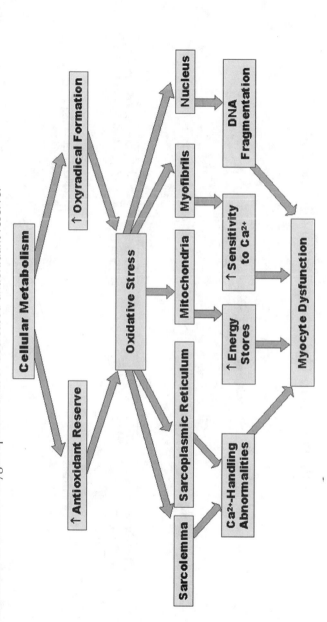

ROS Action on Lipids and Proteins in the Cell[49]

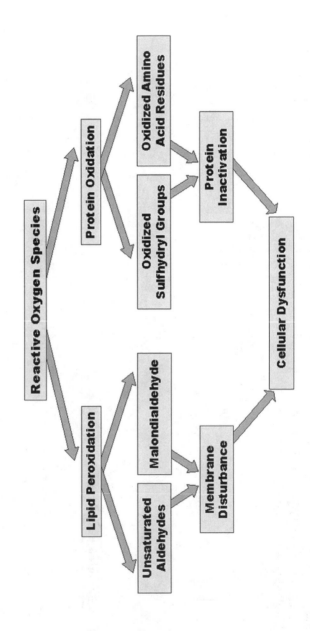

NAD(P)H Oxidase Generates O_2^- via A-II (p22 PHOX)[50,52]

1. Phagocytes or other inflammatory migratory cells
2. Endothelial cells
3. Vascular smooth muscle cells
4. Mesangial cells
5. Podocytes
6. Proximal kidney tubules
7. Adventitial fibroblasts

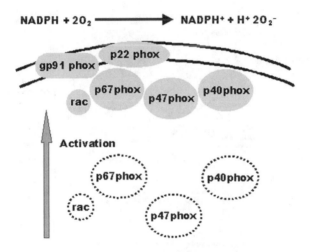

The subunits rac, p67phox, p47phox, and p40phox reside under normal conditions in the cytosol and associate with the membrane-bound gp91phox/p22phox subunits only after activation. Although differences exist between this depicted multienzyme from neutrophils and the NAD(P)H oxidase from nonphagocytic cells, there are several common subunits, including p22phox, that play an important role in A-II-mediated reactive oxygen species generation. A-II stimulates transcription of p22phox subunits in various cells, providing one mechanism for how the vasopeptide may activate NAD(P)H-oxidase.

O_2^- and $O_2^{\bullet-}$ Signal Transduction Pathways[48,50]

Mitochondrial respiration accounts for most of the superoxide generated in a cell with leakage sites at complex I and at ubisemiquinone. The steady-state concentration of superoxide is kept low in all compartments by SODs. The low levels of the radical remaining may modulate various kinases, or may activate transcription factors to effect gene regulation in the nucleus. It is interesting to speculate on the existence of a cell surface receptor for superoxide(R), which might transduce various responses within the cell by means of kinase activation. There is presently no direct evidence for such a receptor.

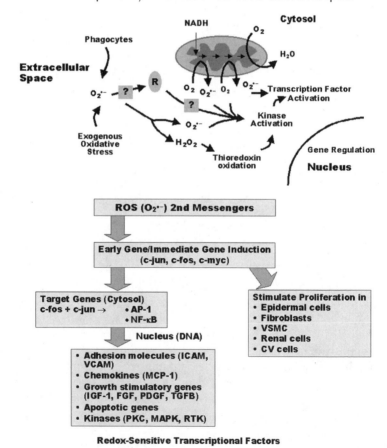

Redox-Sensitive Transcriptional Factors

The Nuclear Factor-κB System of Transcription Factors[3]

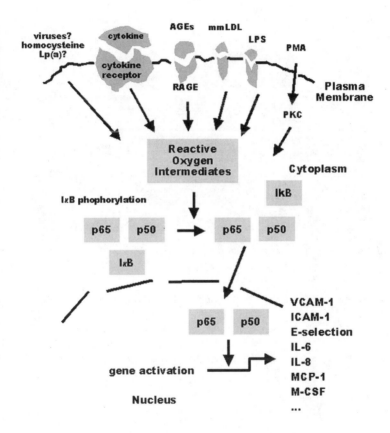

See previous pages for key to abbreviations.
RAGE, receptor-advanced glycosylation end-products; LPS, lipoprotein polysaccharides; PKC, protein kinase C.

ROS and NO[12]

Some of the complex interactions involved in regulating the balance of nitric oxide (NO) and superoxide (O_2-) within the vasculature.

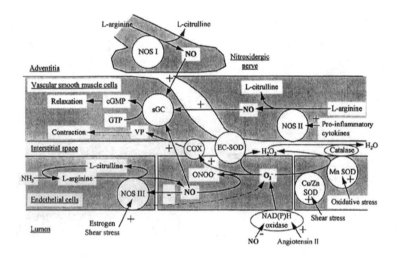

NOS I, neuronal NOS; NOS II, inducible NOS; NOS III, endothelial NOS; EC-SOD, extracellular superoxide dismutase; Mn SOD, manganese SOD; Cu/Zn SOD, copper/zinc SOD; sGC, soluble guanylate cyclase; ONOO_, peroxynitrite; H_2O_2, hydrogen peroxide; GTP, guanosine 5'-triphosphate; COX, cyclooxygenase; VP, vasoconstrictor prostanoids.

Angiotensin and Oxidative Stress in Essential Hypertension[54]

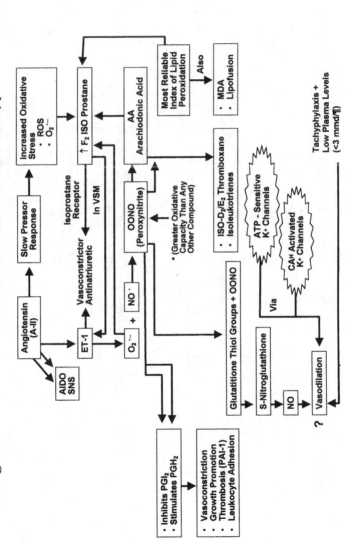

136

Activation of Fast and Slow Intracellular Signaling of A-II[54]

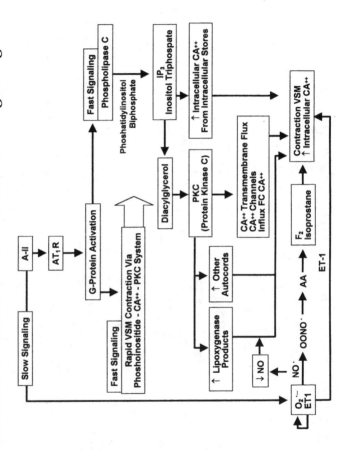

Role of ROS on Hypertension and Hyperlipidemia and Atherosclerosis[50]

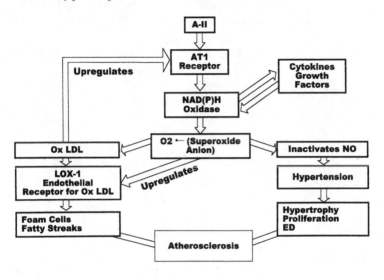

Lox-1 Gene and Receptor
Common Link: HBP, HLP, DM

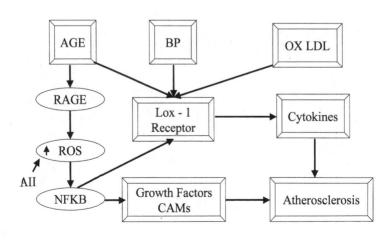

Discussion

The Lox-1 receptor (Lox-1-R) is stimulated by oxidized LDL (oxLDL), advanced glycosylation end-products (AGEs) seen in diabetes mellitus, and by elevated BP. In addition, AGE stimulates the AGE receptor (RAGE), which increases ROS and activates nuclear factor kappa-beta (NFKB), which also stimulates Lox-1-R. Production of cytokines, growth factors, CAMs, and other mediators of atherosclerosis is the final result.

Oxidative Stress and CV Disease: Treatment[49]

The defense mechanisms agains oxidative stress involved in the different stages of cardiac dysfunction to heart failure.

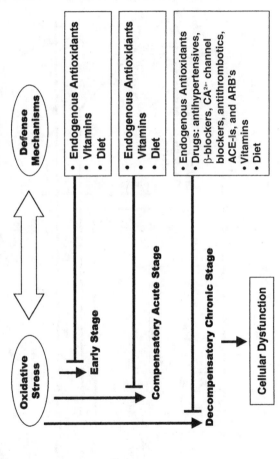

ACE-I, angiotensin converting enzyme inhibitor.

Oxidative Stress and Treatment: Nitrate Tolerance[51,52]

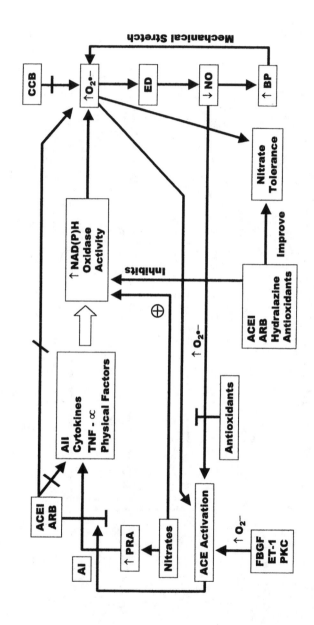

Summary
Oxidative Stress and Cardiovascular Disease

Oxidative stress is the predominant mediator of numerous diseases and is markedly increased in atherosclerosis, hypertension, hyperlipipemia, NIDDM, acute ischemic syndromes, CHD, ischemic reperfusion injury, and CHF. Increased production of ROS or decreased antioxidant reserve creates a pro-oxidant imbalance in the vascular system. ROS induces lipid peroxidation, protein oxidation, carbohydrate oxidation, DNA oxidation and damage, and other organic molecule oxidation.

ROS consists of intracellular signal transduction systems and modulators of transcriptional pathways. ROS and O_2 neutralize NO and its favorable cardiovascular effects.

The antihypertensive drugs most effective in reducing ROS are ARBs, ACEIs and CCBs. Combinations of these three classes of drugs will effectively reduce the production and/or activity of ROS. This nonhypertensive effect improves endothelial dysfunction and vascular smooth muscle dysfunction independent of BP reduction. This adds another dimension to improving vascular health.

Chapter 12

Arterial Compliance

Vascular Compliance: Introduction and Overview[69,70,72,73,74,78]

➤ Function and structural alterations of the arterial wall precede atherosclerosis and cardiovascular events. Endothelial dysfunction is the earliest marker of these changes.[78]

➤ Pharmacological treatment of hypertension has reduced CVA to predicted levels but CHD reduction has been sub-optimal. This **"CHD GAP"** may be due to lack of therapeutic response in improving:

1. Endothelial dysfunction (ED)
2. Arterial compliance (AC)
3. Concomitant risk factors
4. Hemodynamic and hypertension dysfunction

➤ ED affects AC via NO

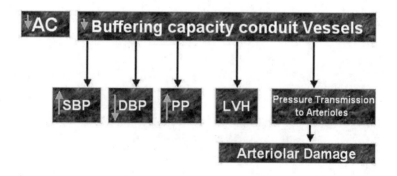

Vascular Compliance: Definitions[78,79,80]

- Compliance = dV/dP (arterial dimension change)

- Stiffness = Eh/2R

- Distensibility = $\dfrac{\Delta\ V/V}{\Delta\ P}$ (fractional change artery caliber)

- Pulse Wave Velocity (PWV) = $\dfrac{\text{Distance}}{\text{Time}}$ (PWV $\dfrac{1}{AC}$)

- Stress = $\dfrac{\text{W tension}}{\text{W thickness}}$ (P x r)

- Strain = $\dfrac{\Delta\ \text{arterial caliber}}{\text{Stress}}$

- Elastic Modulus (EM) = $\dfrac{\Delta\ \text{stress}}{\Delta\ \text{strain}}$

The Vocabulary of Arterial Compliance

Compliance	• Ability of arteries to store temporarily the blood volume ejected with each heartbeat in order to maintain a more continuous tissue perfusion; a measure of this buffering function • A change in area, volume, or diameter for a given change in pressure • Dependent on vessel geometry and mechanical properties • Influenced by structural and functional elements
Distensibility	• Elasticity of the vessel • A change-in-area to a change-in-pressure relationship, at a given starting volume • Independent of vessel geometry

Van Bortel LMAB et al. Am J Cardiol. 1995;76;46E-49E. Cohn JN. Am J Cardiol. 1995;76:34 E-37E. Glasser SP et al. Am J Hypertens. 1997; 10:1175-1189. McVeigh GE, Izzo JL, Black HR, eds. Hypertension Primer. 2nd ed. From the Council on High Blood Pressure Research. American Heart Association. Philadelphia, Lippincott Williams & Wilkins; 1999:327-329.

Vascular Compliance: Arterial Structure

Artery Structure Determines Vascular Stiffness/Compliance

- Intima: Endothelium
                     Subendothelium

- Media: Elastic SM fibers
                     Protein matrix: elastin + collagen
                     Internal elastic membrane

- Adventitia: Fibrous tissue (strong vessel shape large arteries)

Vascular Compliance: Artery Types[69,70,72,73,74,78]

- Conduit (Capacitive): C1 (store blood in systole) (buffer)
  (thin endothelium with thick elastin and collagen) ↓VSM

- Branch (Oscillatory): C2 (pressure oscillations/reflected waves)
  (intermediate structure)

- Arterioles (Resistance): C2 (control blood flow)
  VSM + endothelium primarily with minimal elastin or
  collagen)
  NO dependent.
  Early marker vascular disease (HBP, HLP, DM)

Endothelium role is greatest in thin wall vessels (oscillatory and
resistance). ED earlier and greatest in C-2 vessels.

Arterial Vessel Structure is Heterogeneous

Variables	Elastic/Muscular Conduit Arteries (C1)	Relfecting Sites (C2)	Arterioles (C2)
Elastin	+++	++	+
Collagen	+++	++	+
Smooth muscle	+	++	+++
Endothelium	+	++	++++

Illustration of Circulatory System

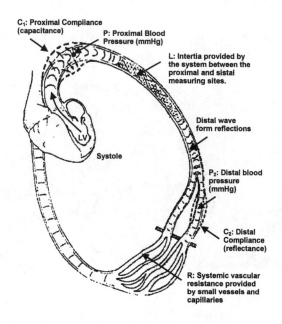

C₁: Proximal Compliance (capacitance)

P: Proximal Blood Pressure (mmHg)

L: Intertia provided by the system between the proximal and sistal measuring sites.

Distal wave form reflections

Systole

P₂: Distal blood pressure (mmHg)

C₂: Distal Compliance (reflectance)

R: Systemic vascular resistance provided by small vessels and capillaries

Buffering System of Vasculature[73]

- In systole there is rapid infusion of SV
  - 20 – 30% is forward flow
  - 70 – 80% is stored in large conduit (capacitive) arteries,
    then released to periphery during diastole

- Converts pulsatile flow in aorta to continuous flow in capillaries (Windkessel effect)

- Loss of buffering with ↓ AC causes reduced continuous flow but increased pulsatile flow to precapillary and capillary vasculature inducing small vessel damage, end organ dysfunction and damage (↑↑PWV)

- Out of phase propagation of flow and pressure waves.
  - Pressure wave faster and distorted
  - Reflected wave
  - Augmentation index (systole)

The Normal, Compliant Vessel vs. the Noncompliant Vessel

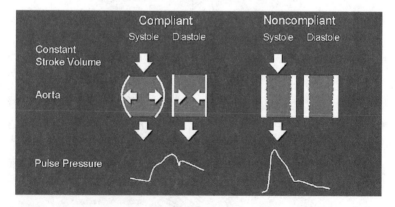

Modified from Bentley DW, Izzo JL. J Am Geriatr Soc. 1982;30:352-359.
Modified from Kelly R. Circulation. 1989;80:1652-1659. Modified from
McVeigh GE et al. Hypertension. 1999;33:1392-1398.

Arterial Blood Pressure Waveform[71]

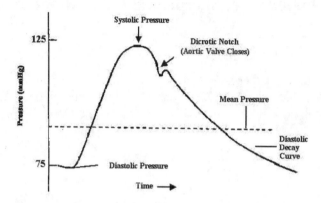

An arterial pressure pulse waveform with the limits of the pressure excursion over the cardiac cycle marked. Systolic pressure represents the peak pressure attained while diastolic pressure represents the trough occurring during the cardiac cycle.

Arterial Compliance and Pulse Contour Analysis

"A reduced systemic compliance that can be derived from analysis of the pulse contour is regarded as the best clinical index of impaired pulsatile arterial function and may mark the presence of early vascular damage."

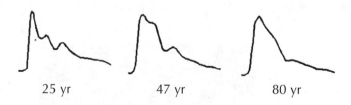

From McVeigh GE et al. Hypertension. 1999;33:1392-1398, with permission.

Arterial Compliance, Resistance, and Impedance: Sharpening the Distinctions

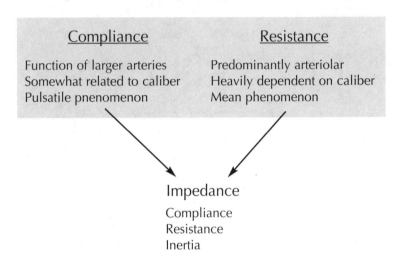

Compliance	Resistance
Function of larger arteries	Predominantly arteriolar
Somewhat related to caliber	Heavily dependent on caliber
Pulsatile pnenomenon	Mean phenomenon

Impedance
Compliance
Resistance
Inertia

Biphasic Behavior of Artery: Collagen and Elastin[73]

- ◆ Nonlinear relationship of arterial wall stiffness related to:
  1. Vascular smooth muscle hypertrophy (VSMH)
  2. Extracellular matrix (ECM)
  3. Blood pressure (BP)

- ◆ Collagen and elastin dependency/properties

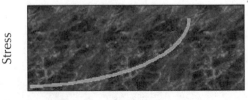

Stress

Strain

Vascular Remodeling[69]

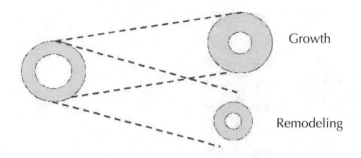

Growth

Remodeling

Vascular Remodeling[108]

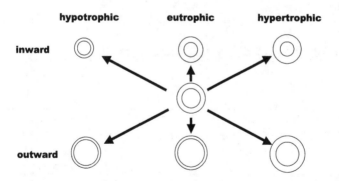

hypotrophic   eutrophic   hypertrophic

inward

outward

How remodeling can modify the cross-sections of blood vessels. The starting point is the vessel at the center. Remodeling can be hypertrophic (e.g., increase of cross-sectional area, vessels in right column), eutrophic (no change in cross-sectional area, vessels in center column), or hypotrophic (e.g., decrease of cross-sectional area, vessels in left column). These forms of remodeling can be inward i.e., reduction in lumen diameter, vessels in top rows) or outward (i.e., increase in lumen diameter, vessels in bottom row).

Vascular Remodeling[69]

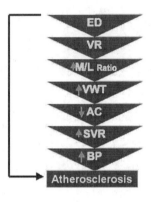

(Endothelial Dysfunction)

(Vascular Remodeling)

(Media / Lumen Ratio)

(Vascular Wall thickness)

(Arterial Compliance)

(Systemic Vascular Resistance)

(Blood Pressure)

Arterial Changes Characterizing Hypertension

Decreased	Increased
Arterial-wall compliance	Media-to-lumen ratio
Endothelium-dependent relaxation	Size of smooth muscle cells
Elastin-to-collagen ratio	Extracellular matrix
Blood flow	Intimal thickening

Plante GE. Can J Cardiol. 1994;10(suppl D):25D-29D. Gibbons GH, Dzau VJ. N Engl J Med. 1994;330:1431-1438. Chobanian AV. Hypertension. 1990;15:666-674. Modified from Ross R. N Engl J Med. 1999;340:115-126.

ACE Inhibition Normalizes Media to Lumen Ratio in the Human Resistance Artery

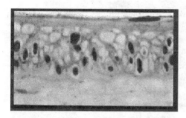 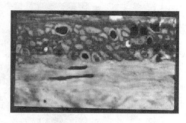

Longitudinal section of resistance artery wall from patient with previously untreated essential hypertension.

Similar section from the same patient after 1 year of perindopril treatment.

Patient was treated with perindopril. From Mulvany MJ, with permission.

Measuring Arterial Compliance (Stiffening)

Method	Measured
Pulse pressure	Predominantly large-artery compliance
Pulse wave velocity	Segmental arterial compliance
Pulse contour analysis	Large- and small-artery compliance
Stroke volume/pulse pressure ratio	Total arterial compliance
Magnetic resonance imaging	Regional aortic compliance
Transcutaneous echo-tracking	Regional aortic compliance

Modified from McVeigh GE. In: Izzo JL, Black HR, eds. Hypertension Primer. 2nd ed. From the Council on High Blood Pressure Research. American Heart Association. Philadelphia, Lippincott Williams & Wilkins; 1999:327-329. Joint National Committee on Prevention, Detection, Evaluation, and Treatment of High Blood Pressure. Arch Intern Med. 1997;157:2413-2446.

The Arterial System and the "Windkessel" Concept: An Historical Association

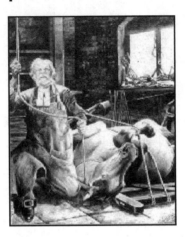

In 1733, Reverend Stephen Hales dramatically demonstrates the first blood pressure device by measuring the BP in the neck of a horse.

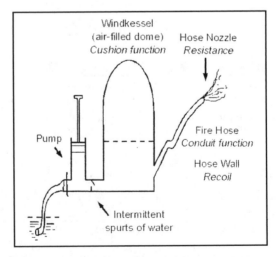

And in 1899, Otto Frank further develops Hales' analogy, likening the arterial circulation's ability to cushion the LV ejection volume to the Windkessel above.

The Modified Windkessel:
Electrical Model for Arterial Circulation

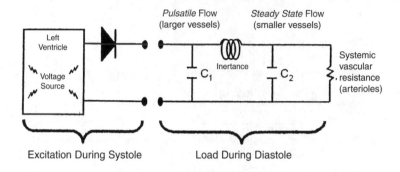

C_1=large-artery compliance, C_2=small-artery compliance.
Modified from Finkelstein SM, et al. Hypertension. 1988;12:380-387.

Arterial Compliance: Measurement[72]

Noninvasive Applanation Tonometry (CAPWA)[72]
(Computerized Arterial Pulse Waveform Analysis)

- Synthesize central pressure waveform from the brachial or radial waveform
- Central hemodynamics improves : Diagnosis, Monitoring, Prognosis
- Index of wave augmentation
    - + Arterial stiffness   + Wave reflection
    - + Vascular load   + Coronary perfusion
- Evaluate therapy
  Central vs peripheral pressure discrepancies
- ↑ PWV correlates with ↑ 24 hour HR (esp. after age 50)
- PWV is independent risk factor for CVD in HBP[96]

Vascular Wall Function and CVD and Hypertension[70,96]

1. Concept of risk marker vs. risk contributor[70]
   Blood pressure is both

2. BP as risk marker

- SBP: ↓ C_1 compliance, ↑ LVH, ↓ aortic storage capacity, ISH, ↑ CHD, CVA, renal risk >> DBP
- DBP ◆ ABM - 24 hour
- Nocturnal BP dipping
- PP: advanced structural changes in conduit artery with ↑ PP, ↑ SBP always is ↑ PP = ↑ CVD
  PP is marker - may be contributor
- PWV is independent CVD risk

Distal Arterial Compliance and CV Outcome

- 419 eligible subjects—proximal (C_1) and distal (C_2) compliance measured at baseline by radial artery pulse contour analysis
- 1- to 7-year follow-up (contacted and returned questionnaires)
- End points: MI, stroke, TIA, angina, coronary or peripheral revascularization, coronary artery or peripheral bypass graft, death

Occurrence of Events as a Function of
Baseline Arterial Compliance*

Variable	Odds Ratio	95% CI Lower	95% CI Upper	p Value
C2	0.67	0.53	0.84	<0.01
Age	1.04	1.02	1.05	<0.001

For each 0.02mm Hg of lowered C_2, there is an approximately 33% increase in the odds ratio for events.

*C1 was associated with age but not outcome. Grey E et al. Am J Hypertens. 2000;13(pt 2). Abstract. Presented at the 15th Scientific Meeting of the American Society of Hypertension.

Arterial Compliance: Structure/Function: Treatment[69,75]

Human trials with gluteal artery biopsies to assess vascular wall structure and function

➤ Correct both structure and function
Increase small artery diameter, increase arterial compliance, decrease media/lumen ratio, decrease SVR and BP remodeling of arterioles
- ◆ ACEI (best)
- ◆ ARB
- ◆ CCB
➤ Correct function (equal ↓BP), no structure change
(No change on ED, AC, M/L ratio, arterial diameter)
- ◆ Diuretic
- ◆ Beta blocker
➤ Nitroglycerin[82,84,93]
- ◆ ↑AC (C-1)
- ◆ ↓PWV
- ◆ No change SVR, distensibility, EM
- ◆ ↓SBP, ↓PP (10%), no change DBP

Antihypertensive Drug Effects on Vascular Remodeling in Humans[108]

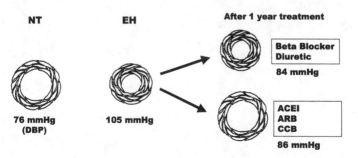

NT	EH	After 1 year treatment
		Beta Blocker Diuretic 84 mmHg
76 mmHg (DBP)	105 mmHg	**ACEI ARB CCB** 86 mmHg

Effects on Structural and Functional Changes in Compliance Appear to Vary Among Antihypertensive Drug Classes*

Drug Class	No. of Agents Tested	No. of Studies	No. of Patients	Increase in Arterial Compliance Yielded
ACE inhibitors†	8	15	~273	With Agents studied (perindopril was most used agent)††
Calcium channel blockers	8	11	~150	With agents studied
β-blockers	7	10	~326	With none, except "vasodilating" β-blockers
Diuretics	4	5	~75	Little effect beyond that associated with ↓BP (an attempt was made methodologically to separate pressure-dependent from direct effects)

*Studies are primarily cross-sectional and short term. Thus, these studies can only be used for information regarding directional effects and by and large cannot distinguish functional from structural changes. The number of published studies using nitrovasodilators, α-blockers, and clonidine are too few for inclusion.

†Certain studies of ACE inhibitors included evaluation of biopsy-demonstrated improvement in vascular remodeling.

††Of the ACE-inhibition studies cited, perindopril was the agent tested in the greatest total number of patients.

Perindopril is the only ACE inhibitor with FDA-approved labeling that cites an increase in the compliance of large arteries.

Modified from Glasser SP et al. J Clin Pharmacol 1998;38:202-212.

Acute Drug Effects on Compliance

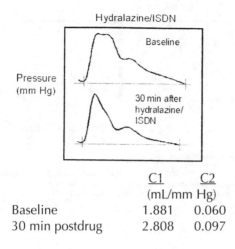

	C1	C2
	(mL/mm Hg)	
Baseline	1.881	0.060
30 min postdrug	2.808	0.097

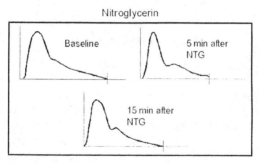

	C1	C2
	(mL/mm Hg)	
Baseline	2.172	0.052
5 min postdrug	2.103	0.104
15 min postdrug	2.443	0.042

ISDN=irosorbide dinitrate, NTG=nitroglycerin.
Reprinted from Cohn JN et al. Hypertension. 1995;26:503-508.
S.P. Glasser, MD, personal communications, 2000.

Apoptosis, CV Remodeling: Treatment[77]

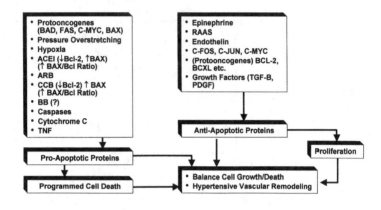

Discussion

Apoptosis, or programmed cell death, is crucial to maintaining vascular health, integrity and a balance between cell growth and death. Forces that interrupt apoptosis (anti-apoptotic), such as the RAAS, induce proliferation, abnormal cell growth, improper balance, and vascular remodeling with a reduction in arterial compliance due to structural and functional changes in the vascular smooth muscle.

Antihypertensive Drug Effects on Apoptosis[81]

ACEI and CCB (amlodipine)

- ↓aortic CSA and ↓BP
- ↑ DNA laddering (pixels /ug NA)
- ↑ BAX/Bcl-2 ratio
  - ↑ BAX gene expression → apoptotic
  - ↓ Bcl-2 gene expression → anti-apoptotic
- Promote through apoptosis regression in vascular growth in hypertension

Antihypertensive Drug Effects on Apoptosis[81]

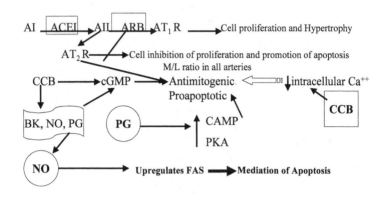

Arterial Compliance: Summary

Arterial compliance, defined as a change in dimension in response to a given change in stress, is becoming an increasingly important clinical parameter. Related concepts, such as distensibility, elasticity, and stiffness, and more traditional concepts such as resistance, afterload, and impedance, need to be differentiated from compliance, although they are frequently (inappropriately) used interchangeably. Many studies cannot differentiate between compliance changes due to a drug's effect on blood pressure and those due to a drug's effect on vessel wall integrity. This differentiation is important because a more physiologic therapy, one that benefits pulsatile and nonpulsatile flow, should be of greater clinical benefit than a therapy that only lowers blood pressure. A number of methods have been used to estimate compliance, but to date there is no generally agreed-on best method. There are longitudinal studies that relate abnormal compliance and drug effects to outcome. Patients at risk from a variety of disease states, such as hypertension, diabetes mellitus, and hypercholesterolemia, may benefit from earlier recognition of abnormal compliance. Earlier recognition may lead to interventions that would reduce their risk.

Hypertension: The Disease Continuum

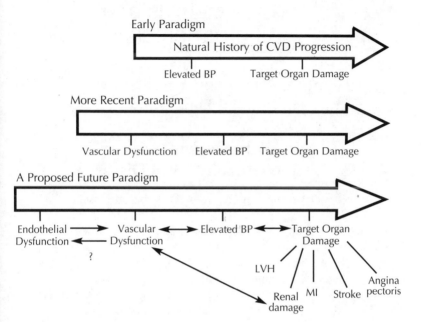

Chapter 13

Hemodynamics and Atherosclerosis

Hemodynamics and Vasculature and Endothelial Function[1,2,88,89]

Atherosclerosis: A Geometrically Focal Disease

➢ Two major hemodynamic forces act on blood vessels

- ◆ Pulsatile Stress: perpendicular pressure/force

- ◆ Shear Stress: parallel pressure/force
  High: longitudinal arteries – low atherosclerosis
  Low: arterial branch points – high atherosclerosis
      (stasis, recirculation, flow separation)
  (High = 12 dyne/cm^2 Low = 4 dyne/cm^2)

➢ Exercise: Mechanisms

- ◆ Increase eNOS/NO

- ◆ Increase cytosolic cu/zn SOD

- ◆ Suppress ACE (↑BK, ↑NO)

- ◆ Induces cyclo-oxygenase 2

➢ Endothelial response is positive or negative with:
   vasoactive agents, antioxidants, growth regulators,
   inflammatory mediators, adhesion molecules, thrombosis

Shear Stress and Endothelial Dysfunction[88]

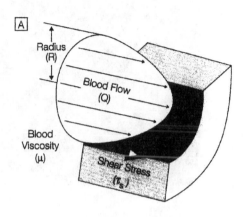

Poiseuille's Law $\quad \tau_s = \dfrac{4\mu Q}{\pi R^3}$

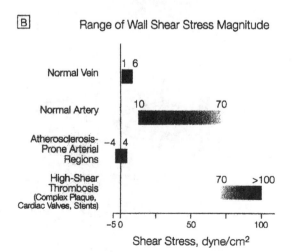

164

Shear Stress and Atherosclerosis[88]

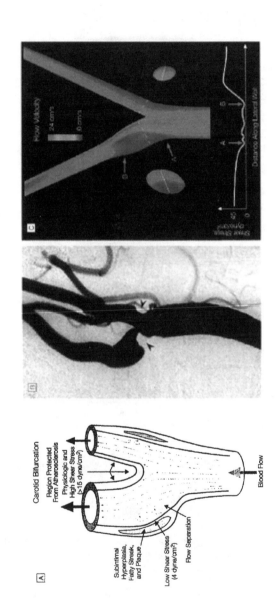

Shear Stress and Endothelial Activation and Dysfunction[88]

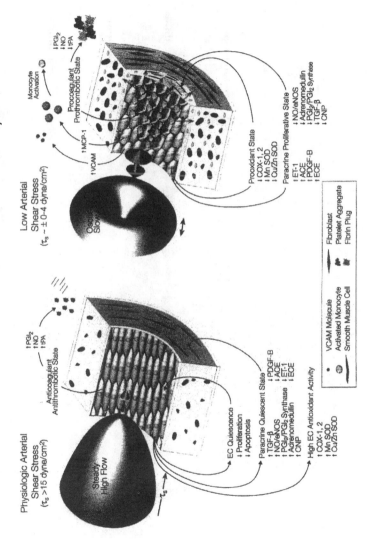

Shear Stress and Atherosclerosis[89]

➢ Multiple Receptors are Activated:

- ◆ Integrins
- ◆ PE CAM
- ◆ Caveolae (NO, G-proteins, TK)
- ◆ TKR (Tyrosine Kinase Receptors)
- ◆ Ion Channels (K^+, Na^+, Cl^-)

↓

➢ Signal Cascades → coordinated and orchestrated
mechanotransduction signaling
crosstalk, feedback and
bi-directional communication

↓

➢ Signal Pathways
Activation TK (Tyrosine Kinases)
Activation SK (Serine Kinases)
Rapid rearrangement of cytoskeleton
Production of NO
Production of ROS

↓

➢ Modulation of Endothelial Gene Expression

Effects of Different Shear Stress Patterns and Magnitude Along the Arterial Tree on Endothelial Cells[89]

Induction:

PGI synthase, connexin43, c-myc, c-fos, c-jun, egr I

PDGF-A, tissue factor, smad 6,7

PDGF-B, TGF-b, b-FGF, HB-EG CNP, COX-2

Thrombomodulin, HO-1, thrombospondin laminin B1, myosin light chain kinase, Mn SOD

ICAM-1, GRO, IL-1, IL-6, IL-8 receptor, tPA, lysyl oxidase, Cu/Zn SOD

Repression:

PAI-1. Endothelin converting enzyme. NADH-dehydrogenase, VCAM-1, Endothelin-1, ACE, thrombomodulin

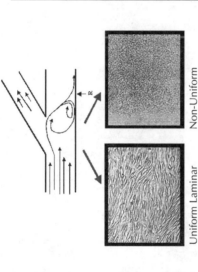

	Uniform Laminar Shear Stress	Non-Uniform Shear Stress
	Gene	Pattern of Regulation
Shear stress Pulsatile	c-fos, c-jun	Induction
	c-myc, PDGF A and B	
Turbulent Oscillatory	TM, b-FGF, PDGF-B HO-1, Cu/Zn SOD, VCAM-1	Induction and Repression
Disturbed LSS	VCAM-1, connexin43	Induction
Shear stress Gradients (In-Vivo)	VCAM-1, PDGF-A	Induction (reduced flow)
	Egr-1	Induction (reduced flow)
	ICAM-1	Induction (increased flow)

While endothelial cells located at straight parts of the arterial tree experience uniform laminar shear stress, at the shoulder of curvatures or bifurcations, these cells are exposed to spatial and temporal shear stress gradients. The morphology of the cells in these areas reflects the forces they are exposed to. Cells that experience uniform laminar shear stress are elongated and aligned in the directions of the flow, while under disturbed shear stress they bear a chaotic morphology. Not only the morphology of the cells differ under these shear stress conditions, but the pattern of gene expression as well. While some of the genes which are induced by uniform laminar shear stress are further induced by disturbed flow (connexin43, egr-1 etc.), VCAM-1 which is repressed by uniform laminar shear stress is induced b disturbed flow. This, suggests that endothelial cells under non-uniform shear stresses are proatherogenic.

Transformation of Endothelial Cell Morphology by Fluid Shear Stress[88]

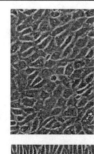

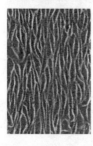

Physiologic Arterial Hemodynamic Shear Stress (τs>15 dyne/cm²)

Low Arterial Hemodynamic Shear Stress (τs ~±0-4 dyne/cm²)

Bovine aortic endothelial cells exposed to physiologic shear stress >15 dyne/cm² (left panel) for 24 hours align in the direction of blood flow while those exposed to low shear stress (right panel) do not (phase contrast; original magnification x 125).

Endothelial Response to Hemodynamic Shear Stress*

	Hemodynamic Shear Stress	
	Physiologic Arterial Magnitude (τs>15 dyne/cm²)	Low Arterial Magnitude (τs~± 0-4 dyne/cm²)
	Fusiform aligned	Polygonal unaligned
Endothelial cell morphology		
Endothelial cell function		
Vasoactive agents		
Vasoconstrictors		
ET-1[102]/ECE[86]	Low	High
ACE[60]	Low	High
Vasodilators		
NO/NO synthase[67-69,81-83]	High	Low
PGI²/PGI² synthase[83-84]	High	Low
CNP[86]	High	Low
Adrenomedullin[87]	High	Low
Antioxidant enzymes		
COX-1, 2[85]	High	Low
Mn SOD[85]	High	Low
Cu/Zn SOD[93]	High	Low
Growth regulators		
Growth factor		
PDGF-B[78,97]	Low	High
PDGF-A[59]	Low	High
Growth inhibitor		
TGF-β[88]	High	Low
Inflammatory mediators		
MCP-1[101]	Low	High
Adhesion molecules		
VCAM-1[100,101,103]	Low	High
Thrombosis/fibrinolysis		
tPA[85,90]	High	Low
TM[89]	Low	High
Endothelial proliferation[78]	Low	High
Endothelial apoptosis[79]	Low	High

*ET-1 indicates endothelin 1; ECE, endothelin-converting enzyme; ACE, angiotensin-converting enzyme; NO, nitric oxide; PGI², prostacyclin; CNP, C-type natriuretic peptide; COX, cyclooxygenase; Mn SOD, manganese-containing superoxide dismutase; Cu/Zn SOD, copper/zinc-containing superoxide dismutase; PDGF-A, B, platelet-derived growth factor A-chain, B-chain; TGF-β, transforming growth factor beta; MCP-1, monocyte chemotactic peptic 1; VCAM-1, vascular cell adhesion molecule 1; tPA, tissue-type plasmino-

Summary
Hemodynamics and Atherosclerosis

The major hemodynamic forces acting on blood vessels are pulsatile stress and shear stress. The endothelial response may be positive or negative depending on intensity, uniformity, location, concomitant biohumoral mediators, and other factors.

Maintenance of physiologic arterial hemodynamic shear stress with antihypertensive medications, as well as regular aerobic exercise of 30 minutes per day, induces vasodilators (eNOS, NO, etc.), reduces vasoconstrictors, increases antioxidant enzymes, and reduces growth factors, inflammatory mediators, adhesion molecules, and thrombotic tendency.

Chapter 14

Systolic, Diastolic and Pulse Pressure

Relationship to Arterial Compliance[79]

➤ "Science, like life, feeds on its own decay. New facts burn old rules; then newly developed concepts bind old and new together into a reconciling law."

William James
The Will to Believe-1896

➤ Old Concept: Diastolic Hypertension
Hypertension is a disease of the arteriolar vessels, with increased vascular tone leading to increased resistance and elevated mean arterial pressure (MAP) and thus DBP.

➤ New Emerging Concept
Hypertension is a disease of large arteries, and arteriolar vessels and arterial compliance reduction leading to increased SBP, PP and DBP initially, but progression to increased SBP, PP and lowered DBP. AC reduction is a cause and target for therapy. Central aortic and brachial artery pressure may differ.

➤ "A man is as old as his arteries."
— Osler

Diastolic, Systolic and PP: History[72,79]

- William Bright diagnosed HBP by "fullness and hardness" of pulse (1820)

- Sphygmomanometer developed by FA Mohomed (1872)

- Diastolic BP is bad (1872-1971) and (1971-2000)

- Systolic BP is good – measures cardiac strength (1872-1971)

- Systolic BP is bad – Kannel et al. Framingham Study
       SBP better predictor than DBP of CHD (1971)
       SBP better predictor than DBP of CVA (1981)

- Isolated systolic hypertension Dustan et al. (1989)

- SBP vs DBP: Rutan et al. (1989) Epidemiology
           SBP predicts CVD better

- SHEP: Systolic Hypertension in Elderly Program
  1991

- STOP 1991 (Swedish Therapy of Old People)

- MRC 1992 (Medical Research Council)

- SYST-EUR 1997 (Systolic Hypertension in Europe Trial)

- Framingham Heart Study 1997

- STOP-2 1999 (Swedish Therapy of Old People–2)

- USA Today and CNN 2000

Systolic, Diastolic and Pulse Pressure: Concepts[72]

♦ SBP > DBP to predict CVD — qualified

♦ PP predicts CVD with absolute superiority in some populations

♦ DBP in elderly if low is associated with ↑CVD

Risk of Cardiovascular Events by Level of Systolic Blood Pressure[90]

Framingham Heart Study: 38-Year Follow-up, Ages 35 to 64 yrs

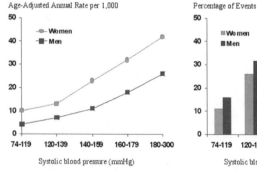

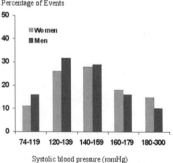

Framingham Heart Study: Subjects aged 35 to 64 years

Risk of Cardiovascular Events by Level of Diastolic Blood Pressure[90]

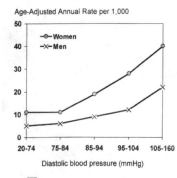

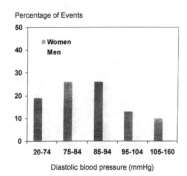

Arterial Pressure Components by Age[85]

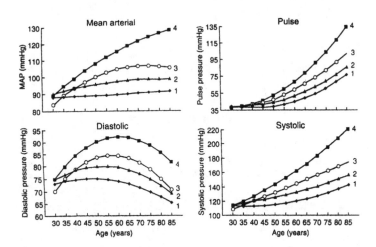

Group averaged individual regression analysis. Curves plotted based on blood pressure-predicted values at 5-year age intervals (age 30-85 years) from least-squares regression equations, developed from individual intercept, slope and quadratic term (curvature), coefficients averaged from individual least-squares mean regressions of each arterial pressure component by age, MAP, mean arterial pressure. Baseline mean systolic blood pressure (SBP) groupings: Group 1, SBP<120 mmHg; Group 2, SBP 120-139 mmHg; Group 3, SBP 140-159 mmHg; Group 4, SBP 160+ mmHg.

Risk of Cardiovascular Events by Type of Hypertension[90]

38-Year Follow-Up

| Types of Hypertension | Age-Adjusted Risk Ratio* | | | |
| | 35-64 yrs. | | 65-94 yrs. | |
	Men	Women	Men	Women
Isolated Diastolic	1.8†	†1.2 ‖	1.2 †	1.6§
Isolated Systolic	2.4§	1.9 ‡	1.9 ‡	1.4 ‡
Combined	2.7%§	2.2%§	2.2%§	1.6%§

* Reference group consists of normotensive persons.
† p <0.05; ‡ p <0.01; § p < 0.001; ‖ p = NS.
Framingham Study: According to Age and Sex

Increase in Risk of Cardiovascular Events per SD Increase in Blood Pressure Parameter[90]

30-Year Follow-Up

| Pressure Component | Standardized Increment in Risk | | | |
| | Men | | Women | |
	35-64 Yrs.	65-94 Yrs.	35-64Yrs.	65-94 Yrs.
Systolic	41%*	51%*	43%*	23%*
Mean Arterial	41%*	44%*	42%*	18%*
Pulse Pressure	29%*	42%*	36%*	22%*
Diastolic	35%*	30%*	33%*	9%†

* p<0.001; † p=NS.
Framingham Study: According to Age and Sex

Age-Adjusted Coronary Heart Disease Death Rates per 10,000 Person-Years[90]

By Level of Systolic Blood Pressure (SBP) and Diastolic Blood Pressure (DBP)

Mean Screened in the Multiple Risk Factor Intervention Trial (21).

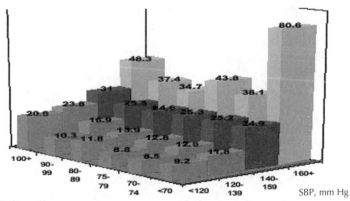

Risk Associated with Increasing Systolic Blood Pressure at Fixed Levels of Diastolic Blood Pressure[95]

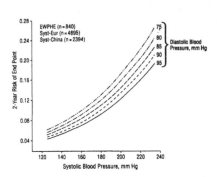

The 2-year probability of a cardiovascular end point was adjusted for active treatment, sex, age, previous cardiovascular complications, and smoking by Cox multiple regression with stratification for trial (European Working Party on High Blood Pressure in the Elderly trial, Systolic Hypertension in Europe Trial, and Systolic Hypertension in China Trial).

Links Between Vascular Mechanics and Epidemiologic Data[72]

The principles of interpretation that relate epidemiologic data to cardiovascular mechanics are as follows:

- Pressure can be separated into two components (steady-pulsatile) that have their own determinants and independent predictive value for cardiovascular events.
- The different patterns of hypertension are due to different mechanisms.
- Pulse waveform is not the same throughout the arterial tree.
- Central pressures are those that are physiologically relevant.

Steady vs. Pulsatile Pressure

- Steady Pressure= <u>MAP</u> (CO x SVR)   ⇑SVR= ⇑MAP
  ↑MAP = Passive increase in SBP + DBP

- Pulsatile Pressure = <u>Impedance</u>
  Impedance ∝ Flow Wave + Pressure Wave

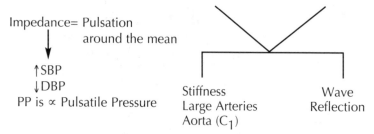

Impedance= Pulsation
          around the mean

↑SBP
↓DBP
PP is ∝ Pulsatile Pressure

Stiffness
Large Arteries
Aorta (C_1)

Wave
Reflection

Types of Hypertension - Mechanisms[72]

BP is a continuous variable and no specific cutoff points should be set in hypertensive or normotensive points.

DBP (Diastolic HBP)

+ ↑DBP with ↑SBP
+ All ages (esp. young)
+ ↑SVR
+ Small ↑arterial stiffness - functional secondary passive over stretch of vascular wall
+ Reflected wave (later) augments DBP most
+ Peripheral pressure > central aortic pressure

SBP (Systolic HBP)

+ ↑SBP with ↓DBP or →DBP
+ Elderly
+ Marked ↑↑arterial stiffness – structural less functional
+ Structural: ↓elastin, ↑collagen, ↑Ca^{++}, ↑ECM
+ Functional: ↓NO, ↑PWV with early wave reflection
+ Reflected wave (earlier) augments SBP most
+ Central and peripheral pressures more equal

Development of Aortic Pressure Abnormalities Due to Age-related Aortic Stiffening[91]

		Normal Aorta (Young Adults)		Stiff Aorta (Older Adults)
1.	Aortic BP (mm Hg)	130 80	Systolic Diastolic	140 70
2.	PWV (m/s)	5.0		10.0
3.	Reflected Wave	Early Diastole		Late Systole
4.	Pulse Wave Shape			
5.	Aortic BP (mm Hg)	130 80	Systolic Diastolic	160 70

1. Increased systolic blood pressure (BP) and decreased diastolic blood pressure due to decreased aortic distensibility.

2. Increased pulse wave velocity (PWV) as a result of decreased aortic distensibility.

3. Return of the reflected primary pulse to the central aorta in systole rather than diastole because of faster wave travel.

4. Change in the shape of the pulse wave because of early wave reflection. Note the reduction in diastolic pressure-time despite the increase in systolic pressure. Horizontal lines indicate systole; vertical lines indicate diastole.

5. The aortic blood pressure resulting from decreased aortic distensbility and early reflected waves.
   *Primary reflected wave. Adapted from reference 18; pulse calibrations added by the authors.

Isolated Systolic Hypertension (ISH)[72]

♦ ↑PWV

♦ ↓AC

♦ ↑Wave Reflection

♦ Treatment
    ACEI
    ARB   Modify wave reflection
    CCB   Decrease central pressure
    Nitrates   No change peripheral pressure

♦ HOPE Trial:
    ACEI independent effects
    BP reduction – measured (3/2 mm Hg)
    Decrease central pressure >> peripheral pressure
        (more than 3/2 mm Hg ?)

Pulse Pressure Facts[72]

♦ PP > 65 mm Hg + HR of 80-100 = deadly combination

♦ CVD by 40-50%/tertile with
    PP < 50 to > 65 mm Hg
    HR < 60 to > 80/min

♦ PP change 10 mm Hg increases   CHD events 13%
                                 CV mortality 20%
                                 Total mortality 15%

♦ PP determined by AC (large arteries) (C-1) + early wave reflection

♦ PP is index of pulsatile load

Changes in Arterial Blood Pressure with Age[72]

As Seen in Major Epidemiological Studies

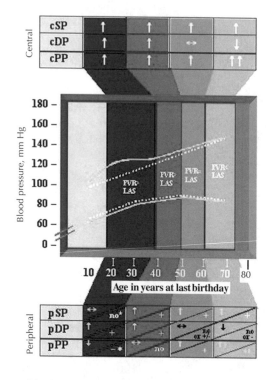

The bottom table shows in the triangulars the predictive value of peripheral blood pressure indices for events. In the graph, solid lines represent published data for brachial pressure; dotted lines indicate predicted pressures in the ascending aorta, based on known differences in brachial pressure amplification with age. The relative contribution of the underlying hemodynamic mechanisms—(increase in peripheral vascular resistance (PVR) or in large artery stiffness (LAS))—is changing progressively from younger to older age. Up arrows indicate increase; down arrows indicate decrease; left/right arrows indicate no change in blood pressure with age. +, Positive; ++, strong positive; -, negative; +/-, weak positive; no, no predictive value. *In males. cDP– central diastolic pressure; cPP– central pulse pressure; cSP– central systolic pressure; pDP–peripheral diastolic pressure; pPP–peripheral pulse pressure; pSP–peripheral systolic pressure.

Conclusions: SBP, DBP, PP and CV Risk[72,85]

◆ Young HBP < 50: DBP best

◆ Middle Age 50-60:   SBP = DBP (50)
                               SBP > DBP (50-60)
                               PP emerges (50-60)

◆ Elderly > 60: PP most important ++
                     SBP important +
                     DBP negative predictor -

Assessment of Endothelial Dysfunction and Subclinical Vascular Disease[5,19]

- ◆ CAPWA: Computerized Arterial Pulse Waveform Analysis (C1+ C2)
- ◆ EBT: Electron Beam Tomography (CAC and CVS): plaque
- ◆ CWIMT: Carotid Wall Intimal-Medial Thickness
- ◆ ABI: Ankle Brachial Index
- ◆ ECHO: LVH and diastolic dysfunction
- ◆ MRI BRAIN: Subclinical ischemic microinfarcts and white matter
- ◆ BA-FMD: Brachial Artery Flow Mediated Dilation
- ◆ Forearm Plethysmography
- ◆ Acetylcholine Infusion
- ◆ PC-MRI Heart: Phase Contrast MRI (plaque burden)
- ◆ IVUS: Intravascular Ultrasound
- ◆ TER A/B: Transcapillary Albumin Escape Rate
- ◆ 24 HR MAU: Microalbuminuria
- ◆ Traditional Risk Factors: BP, Lipids, Glucose, HgA_1C, Homocysteine, etc.
- ◆ Emerging Risk Factors: HS-CRP, CAMS, VWF, tPA/PAI-ratio, ADMA, Adrenomedullin, CSF, MCP-1, Cytokines, Oxidation Products, Insulin, etc.
- ◆ PET-derived myocardial blood flow

Summary
Systolic, Diastolic, and Pulse Pressure

Systolic, diastolic, and pulse pressure are all predictive of cardiovascular and cerebrovascular morbidity and mortality, but the relative importance is age dependent.

In patients below age 50 years, DBP is the best predictor of CV risk. In patients 50 to 60 years of age, PP emerges as more predictive, followed by SBP and then DBP. After age 60, PP is the most important, followed by SBP. The DBP is actually a negative predictor in that a lower DBP predicts a greater CV risk.

Loss of aortic compliance and its buffering capacity increases arterial stiffness, increases PWV, SBP, and PP, and lowers DBP. Thus elevated PP is a marker for significant vascular disease. This is due to increased collagen and loss of elastin in the media of the blood vessel wall.

Antihypertensive drugs, which increase elastin, decrease collagen, and increase aortic compliance, are most likely to reduce SBP and PP. ARBs, ACEIs and CCBs probably do this most effectively.

Chapter 15
Effects of Antihypertensive Drugs on Arterial Compliance

Treatment: Hypertension and Arterial Compliance

ARIC STUDY: Atherosclerosis Risk in Communities Study[83]

Relationship of Arterial Stiffness and Hypertension

> 10,712 men and women
> Age: 45-64 years
> BP > 140/90 mm Hg or use of anti-HBP meds
> Common carotid arterial diameter change with B mode U/S

> Conclusion:
> Hypertension is associated with increased carotid arterial stiffness.
> Adjusted diameter change .33 mm vs .43 mm
> (p < 0.01)

Additional Large Scale Trials re PWV, AC, Central BP[84]
- ASCOT: HBP
- SEARCH: HLP
- FIELD: DM

Antihypertensive Drugs and Vascular Disease/Arterial Compliance[75]

➢ Large Muscular Arteries (Brachial/Radial)
- Change I/M thickness
- Contribute to SVR
➢ Resistance Arteries
- Critical determinants of SVR
- Related to CVA, nephro-angiosclerosis, myocardial ischemia

Cardiovascular Drugs and Arterial Compliance[73,74,75]

➤ Concept

Antihypertensive drugs that vasodilate may affect function and structure. Ideal drug will:
- ◆ Lower BP (hemodynamics) (↓ SVR)
- ◆ Increase AC (structure) (C1 + C2)
- ◆ Reduce VSMC hypertrophy (structure)
- ◆ Improve ED (function)
- ◆ Decrease SBP, DBP and PP (↓ reflected waves)

➤ Surrogate Short-term Human Studies

➤ Supporting Clinical Trials

CAPPP, STOP-2, HOPE, SYST-EUR, HOT, GLASCOW BP CLINIC

Antihypertensive Drugs and Arterial Compliance[73,74,75]

	C1	C2	ED	PWV	M/L Ratio
NP	↑	↑	↓	↓	
NTG	↑↑	↑	↓	↓	
CCB	↑↑	↑	↓	↓	↓
ACEI	↑	↑↑	↓	↓	↓
ARB	↑	↑	↓	↓	↓
Diuretic	→	→	→	→	
BB	→	→	→	→	
∝ B	→	→	→	→	
CAA	→	→	→	→	
DV	→	→	→	→	
VPI	↑	↑	↓	↓	

NP= nitroprusside, NTG= nitroglycerin, CCB= calcium channel blocker, ACEI= angiotensin converting enzyme inhibitor, ARB= angiotensin receptor blocker, BB= beta blocker, ∝ B= alpha blocker, CAA= central alpha agonist, DV= direct vasodilator, VPI= vasopeptidase inhibitor, C1= large artery compliance, C2= small artery compliance, ED= endothelial dysfunction, PWV= pulse wave velocity, M/L ratio= media/lumen ratio of blood vessel.

The Role of Diuretics in Vascular Compliance[74]

Drug	Author (reference)	Technique	No. of Patients	Comparator Therapy	Findings
Thiazide	Levenson et al (37)	PWV	10/HTN	none	unchanged beyond BP
	Breithaupt et al (36)	PWV	17/HTM	cilazapril	cilazapril ↑ VC amiloride HCTZ did not
Amiloride/ HCTZ	Van Bortel et al (26)	echo tracking		perindopril 1	brachial artery no ↑ VC, carotid artery VC
	Levenson et al (37)	PWV	8/HTN	thiazide	cilazapril ↑ VC, amiloride/ HCTZ did not
	Kool et al (33)	echo tracking	20/HTN	perindopril	perindopril ↑ VC> amiloride/HCTZ
Furosemide	Domingo et al (38)	PWV	10 NL/10 CHF	captopril/captopril + furosemide	captopril + furosemide ↑ VC > C > F

PWV, pulse wave velocity; HTN, hypertensive; BP, blood pressure;, increased; VC, vascular compliance; HCTZ, hydrochlorothiazide; CHF, congestive heart failure

The Role of β-Adrenergic Blocking Agents in Vascular Compliance[74]

Drug	Author (reference)	Technique	No. of Patients	Comparator Therapy	Findings
Metoprolol	De Cesaris et al (27)	2D flowmetry	25/HTN	lisinopril	lisinopril ↑ VC, metoprolol did not
	De Luca et al (42)	2D flowmetry	15/HTN	ketasartin	ketasartin ↑ VC, metoprolol did not
Propranolol	Ting et al (19)	ultrasound	79/NT, 79/HTN	various	propranolol did not normalize VC
	Levenson et al (39)	pulsed Doppler	12/HTN		no change in VC
Atenolol	Perret et al (21)	ultrasound	32/NT	lisinopril/nitrendipine	only lisinopril ↑ VC
	De Cesaris (27)	PWV	20/HTN	nicardipine	nicardipine ↑ VC, atenolol did not
	Hayoz et al (28)	echo tracking	32/NT	lisinopril/nitrendipine	only lisinopril ↑ VC
	Kelly et al (41)	PWV	12/HTN	dilevalol	dilevalol ↑ VC, atenolol did not
Medroxalol	Chau et al (14)	2D flowmetry	11/HTN	variety	medroxalol had no effect on VC
Dilevalol	Kelly et al (41)	PWV	12/HTN	atenolol	dilevalol ↑ VC, atenolol did not
Acebutolol	Levenson et al (40)	forearm		variety	acebutolol ↑ VC
Nebivalol	van Merode et al (25)	Doppler	29/HTN	placebo	nebivalol ↑ VC

2D, two-dimensional; HTN, hypertensive;, increased; VC, vascular compliance; NT, normotensive; PWV, pulse wave velocity.

The Effect of Calcium Channel Antagonists on Arterial Compliance[74]

Drug	Author (reference)	Technique	No. of Patients	Treatment	Findings
Nitrendipine	Chau et al (14)	Pulsed Doppler	13/HTN	variety	nitrendipine ↑ VC
	Asmar et al (15)	PWV	17/HTN	placebo	nitrendipine ↑ VC
Lacidipine	Pancera et al (17)	tonometry	18/HTN	placebo	lacidipine ↑ VC
	Salar et al (24)	Doppler flowmetry	10/NT	placebo, double-blind crossover	lacidipine ↑ VC
	Mancia et al (47)	variety	review article	variety	lacidipine ↑ VC
Nifedipine	Shimamoto et al (18)	pulsed Doppler	26 ELD/HTN	lisinopril	lisinopril ↑ VC> nifedipine
	Ting et al (19)	intravascular and tonometry	variety	variety	nifedipine ↑ VC
Nicardipine	De Cesaris et al (20)	2D Doppler flowmetry	20/20/HTN	atenolol	nicardipine ↑ VC>atenolol
Nitrendipine	Perret et al (21)	ultrasound	32/NT	atenolol, lisinopril, placebo	only lisinopril ↑ VC
Isradipine	Wysocki et al (22)		14/HTN	none	isradipine ↑ VC
Diltiazem	Safar et al (24)	Doppler	11/HTN	dihydralazine	diltiazem ↑ VC
Verapamil	van Merode et al (25)	Doppler	19/HTN	placebo	verapamil ↑ VC

HTN, hypertensive; ↑, increased; VC, vascular compliance; PWV, pulse wave velocity; NT, normotensive; ELD, elderly; 2D, two dimensional.

The Effect of Angiotensin-Converting Enzyme Inhibitors on Vascular Compliance[74]

Drug	Author (reference)	Technique	No. of Patients	Treatment	Findings
Lisinopril	De Cesaris et al (27)	2D flowmetry	25/25/HTN NT	metoprolol atenolol/nitrendipine	only lisinopril ↑ VC
	Hayoz et al (28)	echo tracking			lisinopril ↑ VC
	Shimamoto et al (18)	pulsed Doppler	26 ELD/HTN	nifedipine	lisinopril ↑ VC > nifedipine
Trandolapril	De Luca et al (29)	pulsed Doppler	15/HTN	none	trandolapril ↑ VC
	Asmar et al (30)	PWV	24/HTN	placebo	trandolapril ↑ VC in dose-response fashion
Perindopril	London et al (31)	variety	24/ESRD	nitrendipine	perindopril and nitrendipine ↑ VC
	Van Bortel et al (26)	echotracking	not listed	amiloride/HCTZ	perindopril VC > amiloride/HCTZ
	Asmar et al (32)	Doppler and PWV	15/HTN	none	perindopril ↑ VC
	Kool et al (33)	echo tracking	41/HTN	amiloride/HCTZ	perindopril ↑ VC > amiloride/HCTZ
Quinapril	Schartl et al (34)	PWV	15/HTN	none	quinapril ↑ VC
Captopril	Ting et al (19)	intravascular and tonometry		variety	captopril ↑ VC
	Domingo et al (38)	PWV	10 NL/10 CHF	furosemide/ furosemide + captopril	captopril and furosemide + VC > C > F
Fosinopril	Ting et al (19)	intravascular and tonometry		variety	fosinopril ↑ VC
Enalapril	Asmar et al (35)	pulsed Doppler	16/HTN	none	enalapril ↑ VC
Cilazapril	Breithaupt et al (36)	PWV	17/HTN	HCTZ	cilazapril ↑ VC > diuretic

2D, two-dimensional; HTN, hypertensive;, increased; VC, vascular compliance; NT, normotensive; ELD, elderly; PWV, pulse wave velocity; ESRD, end-stage renal disease; HCTZ, hydrochlorothiazide; NL, normal; CHF, congestive heart failure.

Correction of Arterial Structure and Endothelial Dysfunction in Human Essential Hypertension by the Angiotensin Receptor Antagonist Losartan

Ernesto L. Schiffrin, MD, PhD, FRCPC
Jeong Bae Park, MD
Hope D. Intengan, PhD
Rhian M. Touyz, MD, PhD

Circulation 2000; 101:1653-59

Systolic and Diastolic BP of Patients Treated with Losartan or Atenolol for 1 year

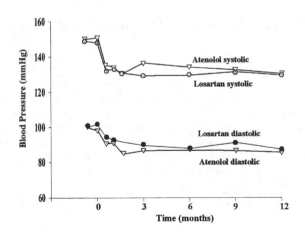

Circulation 2000; 101:1653-59

Change in Individual Media Width to Lumen Diameter (M/L) After 1 Year of Treatment

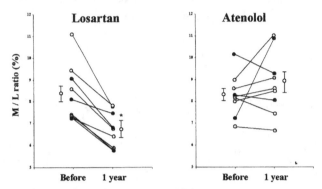

* P < 0.01 vs before treatment and vs atenolol treatment

Circulation 2000; 101:1653-59

Morphologic Characteristics of Resistance Arteries

		Losartan Treatment		Atenolol Treatment	
		Before	1 yr	Before	1yr
External diameter, μm	214 ± 18	124 ± 13	222 ± 21	200 ± 8	191 ± 12
Internal diameter, μm	191 ± 17	184 ± 12	195 ± 18	172 ± 8	164 ± 8
Media width, μm	11.2 ± 1.3	15.2 ± 1.0*	13.4 ± 1.4	14.2 ± 0.5*	14.0 ± 0.5*
M / L r, %	5.9 ± 0.3	8.4 ± 0.4*	6.7 ± 0.3^	8.3 ± 0.3*	8.8 ± 0.5*‡
MCSA, μm²	8035 ± 1708	9835 ± 1194	9404 ± 1817	8362 ± 608	7936 ± 590

MCSA = media Cross-sectional area
* = P<0.05 vs normotensives
^ = P<0.05 vs before treatment
‡ = P<0.05 vs 1-year losartan treatment

Circulation 2000; 101:1653-59

Maximal acetylcholine responses (100μmol/L) of resistance arteries from normotensive subjects and hypertensive patients, in the latter before and after 1 year of antihypertensive treatment.

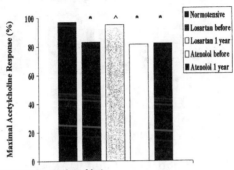

* = P<0.05 vs normotensive subjects
^ = P,0.05 vs losartan group before treatment and vs atenolol treated group

Circulation 2000; 101:1653-59

Conclusions

◆ Treatment with losartan improved structural abnormalities and normalized endothelial function of small arteries from patients with mild to moderate essential hypertension.

◆ None of these effects was found in a parallel group of hypertensive patients treated with atenolol, despite similar BP lowering.

Risk of Cardiovascular Disease in Men Age 40 According to Systolic BP and Risk Profile

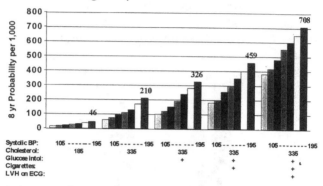

Systolic BP:	105 ----- 195	105 --- 195	105 --- 195	105 ----- 195	105 -------- 195
Cholesterol:	185	335	335	335	335
Glucose intol:			+	+	+
Cigarettes:				+	+
LVH on ECG:				+	+

Framingham, Kannel, WB Am J Cardiol 1976; 37:269-282

LVH and Associated CV Risk

◆ In Framingham and other studies, LV mass and age were the strongest predictors of prognosis.[1,2]

◆ Within 5 years of confirmed LVH, one-third of men and one-fourth of women are dead, usually from coronary disease.[3]

1. Framingham, Levy D et al, N Engl J Med 1990;332:1561-66
2. Koren MJ et al, Ann Intern Med 1991;114:345-52
3. Kannel WB. Prevalence and natural history of ECG LVH. Am J Med 1983;75(suppl 3A):4-11

Excess CV Risk of ECG defined LVH (depending on age and sex) - Framingham Heart Study

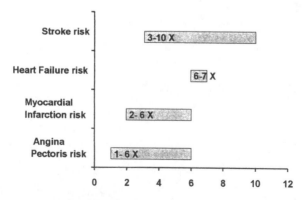

Levy D, Drugs 1998;35(suppl 5):1-5

ECG Determination of LVH in Hypertension

◆ ECG can detect LVH with a high degree of specificity.[1]
◆ LVH detected by either method is associated with a poor prognosis.
◆ ECG may identify an elevation of risk as efficiently or better than echocardiography and at a lower cost.

1. Devereux RB, et al Hypertension 1987;9(suppl II):1169-76

Prevalence of LVH in Hypertension

◆ Prevalence of ECG determined LVH in hypertensive patients in referral centers is approximately 40%, increasing with age.[1-3]

◆ ECG-LVH is approximately 10 times more prevalent in patients with blood pressure > 160/95 mmHg than in normotensive subjects.[4]

1. Savage DD, et al Circulation 1979;59:623-32
2. Devereux RB, et al Hypertension 1982;4:542-31
3. Devereux RB, et al Circulation 1983;68:470-76
4. Kanel WB, et al Ann Intern Med 1969;71:89-105

Possible Gender Issue of LVH in Hypertension

◆ The Glasgow Blood Pressure Clinic reported a prevalence of ECG-LVH of 35% in men and 22% in women with nonmalignant hypertension and a mean age of 50 years, drawn from a high-risk population in western Scotland.

Dunn FG, et al J Hypertens 1990;8:775-82

Hypothetical Effects of AT_2-Receptor Stimulation
Counterbalance Effects of AT_1-Receptor Stimulation

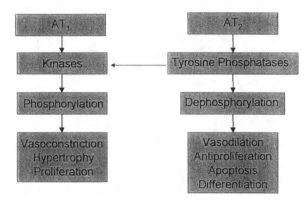

Gasparo M et al, Pharmacol Toxicol 1998;82:257-71

Reversal of LVH in Hypertensive Patients
109 studies of monotherapy for the treatment of hypertension
% change in LV Mass

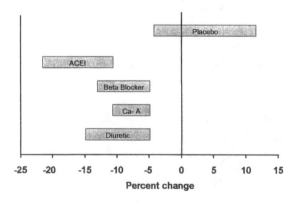

Dahlof B et al, Am J Hypertens 1997;10:705-713
Dahlof B et al, Am J Hypertens 1992;5:95-110

Change in Left Ventricular Mass
109 studies of monotherapy for the treatment of hypertension

	Baseline LVM (g)	Reduction in LVM Δg	%	ΔLVM g / ΔMAP mm Hg
ACE inhibitors	274	45	16.3	2.3
95% CI		23 to 66		1.1 to 3.5
β-Blockers	254	23	9.0	0.9
95% CI		8 to 38		0.07 to 1.7
CCB's	261	27	10.3	1.4
95% CI		12 to 42		0.6 to 2.2
Diuretics	277	21	7.7	1.1
95% CI		-6 to 49		-0.4 to 2.6

Dahlof B, J Hypertens 1993; 11(suppl 3):S29-S35.

% Change in LV Mass
109 studies of monotherapy for the treatment of hypertension

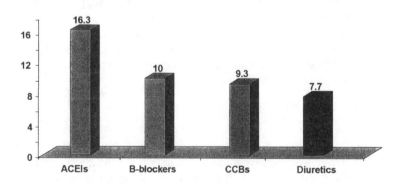

Dahlof B, J Hypertens 1993; 11(suppl 3):S29-S35.

Regression of L V Mass per BP↓
109 studies of monotherapy for the treatment of hypertension

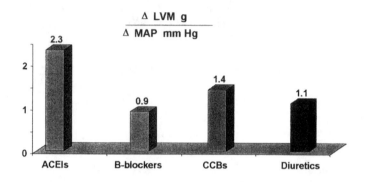

Dahlof B, J Hypertens 1993; 11(suppl 3):S29-S35.

Treatment of Hypertension and LVH

◆ The large Treatment of Mild Hypertension Study (TOMHS) included such a successful nutritional-hygienic regimen that it reduced blood pressure to normal.
◆ Only a small minority of patients had LVH.
◆ The effects of pharmacologic therapies on LVH were limited.
◆ TOMHS suggested no differential between the pharmacologic agents in relation to effects on LVH.

Neaton JD et al, JAMA 1993;270:713-24

◆ A prospective study is needed to determine definitively whether or not antihypertensive therapy that interrupts RAS effects most fully has a greater effect than conventional therapy on reversal of LVH, independent of blood pressure reduction and whether reversal of LVH is connected to a reduction, in CV events.

Devereux RB, et al JAMA 1996;275:1517-18
Devereux RB, et al J Hypertens 1996;14(suppl 2):S95-102

Angiotensin-II Promotes Atherosclerotic Lesions and Aneurysms in Apolipoprotein E-deficient mice

Alan Daugherty, Michael W. Manning, and Lisa A. Cassis

J Clin Invest. 2000; 105:1605-12

Arterial BP Determined Using a Catheter in the Femoral Artery of Anesthetized apoE -/- Mice

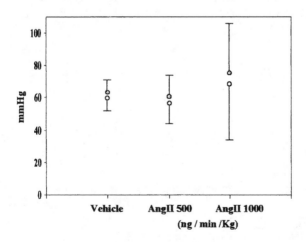

Daugherty A et al, J Clin Invest 2000; 105:1605-12

Systolic and Diastolic Arterial Pressure Measured Using a Femoral Artery Catheter in Groups of Wild-type C57BL/6 Mice

Group	Systolic arterial pressure (mmHg)	Diastolic arterial pressure (mmHg)
Control	85 ± 10	78 ± 10
AngII 500 ng / min / Kg	56 ± 17 (NS)	48 ± 17 (NS)
AngII 1,000 mg / min / Kg	53 ± 9 (NS)	40 ± 7 (NS)

% of Intimal Area Covered by Grossly Discernible Atherosclerotic Lesions in the Thoracic Region

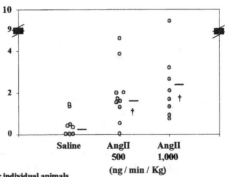

Circles = values for individual animals
Bars = Means for the groups
† = Statistical difference of $p>0.05$ from the control group

Daugherty A et al, J Clin Invest 2000; 105:1605-12

Aneurysms Formed in the
Abdominal Aorta of apoE -/- Mice

Aorta on Right:
  apoE -/- mouse infused with AngII
  1,000 ng/min/Kg for 28 days

Aorta on Left:
  age and gender matched
    apoE -/- mouse
  infused with vehicle for 28 days

Daugherty A et al, J Clin Invest 2000; 105:1605-12

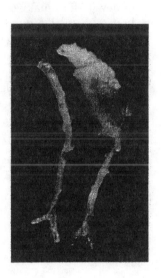

Discussion

◆ After 28 days of Ang II infusion, there were several changes in vascular pathology, including:
  ◆ an increase in the extent of atherosclerosis
  ◆ a change in the nature of lesions and adventitial tissue underlying lesions
  ◆ the formation of large abdominal aortic aneurysms
◆ Medial hypertrophy was noted in the aortas of both apoE -/- and apoE +/+ mice
◆ Ang II provoked marked proinflammatory responses in the perimedial area, manifest as an accumulation of macrophages at the external elastic lamina.

Discussion

◆ The most marked change in artherogenesis was the formation of new lesions that were adjacent to the mature fibrolipid lesions that had formed in the apoE -/- mice
  ◆ A prominent feature of these lesions was the presence of a large number of lymphocytes
◆ Infusion of Ang II into apoE -/- mice promoted the appearance of blood clots and tissue remodeling surrounding an area of marked adventitial hypertrophy. The complex morphology of the aneurysms formed in response to Ang II occurred in the absence of a measureable increase in BP.

Conclusion

◆ Infusion of Ang II into apoE -/- mice with established atherosclerosis leads to augmented lesion formation and the development of abdominal aorta aneurysms
◆ Inhibition of Ang II with ARBs can reduce aortic aneurysm formation.

Daugherty A et al, J Clin Invest 2000; 105:1605-12

Summary
Effects of Antihypertensive Drugs on Arterial Compliance

Numerous studies have demonstrated superiority of ARBs, ACEIs and CCBs on the structure and function of the blood vessel through both BP-dependent and BP-independent mechanisms. These drugs improve arterial compliance.

ARBs improve C1, C2, and EDV1 and reduce ED, PWV, and M/L ratio. ACEIs have an antiatherosclerotic effect in experimental animals.

CCBs improve C1 and C2, and reduce ED, PWV and M/L ratio. CCBs have an antiatherosclerotic effect in experimental animals.

Diuretics and beta blockers, when compared directly to ARBs, ACEIs and CCBs in these studies, do not improve C1, C2, ED, PWV, or M/L ratio. Despite equal BP reductions, the structure and function of the blood vessel remains abnormal.

Treatment of Hypertension: New Approach Based on Vascular Biology

Antihypertensive Drugs[75]

Experimental evidence indicates that antihypertensive drugs decrease morbidity and mortality outcomes (CVD) independent of BP reduction via improved vascular remodeling (↓ED and ↑AC)

New Treatment approach

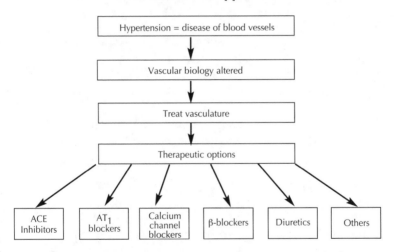

- Hypertension as a disease of the endothelium.
- Vascular biology is altered, and the logical therapy is to improve vascular health and function.
- The role of therapy with ARBs, ACEIs and CCB is now more prominent as they improve endothelial dysfunction, arterial compliance and lower BP. The optimal goal is no longer simply BP reduction.

Treatment of Endothelial Dysfunction[8,9,13]

- ◆ Restore NO Bioavailability
  HBP: CCB, ACEI, ARB
  HLP: Statins
  　　　Fibrates

- ◆ Anti-Lipid Therapy: Statins
  ($\downarrow$ADMA, $\uparrow G_1$CRC, $\downarrow AT_1R$, $\uparrow$ENOS/NO)
  ($\downarrow$OX LDL, EDV, $\downarrow$BP, $\downarrow$ROS, $\downarrow O_2$)

- ◆ Omega 3 PUFA (DHA > EPA): cell membranes

- ◆ Monounsaturated fats

- ◆ Antioxidants: C, E, selenium, NAC, etc.

- ◆ L-Arginine supplements

- ◆ Potassium ($\downarrow$VSMC migration/proliferation, $\downarrow$PDGF,
  $\uparrow$NA/K ATPase, $\uparrow Ca^{++}/Na^{++}$ exchange)

- ◆ Exercise

- ◆ ASA: platelets

- ◆ Antibiotics (?) ($\downarrow$CRP, $\downarrow$IL-6, $\downarrow$TNF)
  Academic, Wizard, ACES

- ◆ ERT in postmenopausal women (or SERMs)

- ◆ Biopterin

- ◆ Reduce homocysteine (folate, B_6, B_{12})

CCB and Endothelial Dysfunction: Treatment[6,9,27,67]

- Counteracts A-II via ↑ in NO bioavailability
- Counteracts ET-1
- Increases eNOS and NO
- Antioxidant (membrane lipid) (amlodipine)
  (↓ROS, ↓O_2)
- Enhances EDHF
- Interferes with cyclooxygenase-derived contracting factors
- ↑ EDV
- Endothelial cell cytoprotection (↓cytokines, ↓CAMs) (amlodipine)
- Modifies of VCMC membrane defect (amlodipine)
- Inhibits VSMC proliferation and migration (amlodipine)
- Inhibits ACAT in macrophages (amlodipine)
- Inhibits cholesterol esterification and oxidation of LDL via lipid peroxide (amlodipine)
- Decreases insulin resistance
- ↑ AC, ↑ C_1AC, ↑ C_2AC, ↓PP, ↑ AD, ↓ASI, ↓PWV, ↓AGI
- ↓ Atherosclerosis
- Anti-platelet effect
- Inhibits tissue necrosis factor (amlodipine)
- Inhibits platelet-derived growth factor (amlodipine)
- Decrease media/lumen ratio (MLR)
- Decrease xanthine oxidase and catalase (amlodipine)
- Decrease βFGF
- Decrease leukotrienes
- Decrease thromboxane B_2
- Decrease fibrinogen

AGI = augmentation index
AD = aortic distensibility
ASI = aortic stiffness index
βFGF = beta fibroblastic growth factor

ACEI and Endothelial Dysfunction: Treatment[6,9,27,34,67]

- ↑ BK
- ↑ NO
- ↑ EDHF
- ↓ Vasopressin
- ↓ ET-1
- ↑ PGI-2
- ↑ Enkephalins
- ↑ EDV
- ↓ CAMS
- ↓ PAI-1 and ↑t-PA (↑ Fibrinolysis)
- ↓ Growth Factors and VSMH
- ↓ ROS/O_2
- ↑ AC_1, ↑ C_1AC, ↑ C_2AC, ↓PWV, ↑ AGI, ↓ASI, ↓PP, ↓AD, ↓ASI
- ↓ Plaque Rupture
- Angiogenesis (myocardial)
- ↓ Atherosclerosis
- ↓ Platelets Effects
- ↑ Ang 1-7
- ↓ Ang II – transient
- ↓ Microalbuminuria (MAU) and proteinuria
- ↓ MLR
- ↓ Fibrinogen

Potency of ACE Inhibitors in Plasma and Tissue (RIB Studies)

Plasma		Tissue
Quinaprilat (400)	High	Quinaprilat (33)
Cilazaprilat (28)		Benazeprilat (27)
Benazeprilat (17)		Perindoprilat (17)
Fosinoprilat (14)		Ramiprilat (11)
Ramiprilat (12)		Lisinopril (6)
Lisinopril (5)		Enalaprilat (2.3)
Enalaprilat (5)		Fosinoprilat (1.7)
Captopril (1)	Low	

Adapted from Fabris B, et al. Br J Pharmacol. 1990:100:651-655.
Fabris B, et al. J Cardiovasc Pharmacol. 1990;15(suppl 2):S6-S13.
Johnston C1, et al. J Hypertens. 1989;7 (suppl 5):S11-S16.

Content points:
- ◆ Radioligand inhibitor binding (RIB) studies demonstrate a wide range of ACE binding affinity among the available ACE inhibitors.

- ◆ Quinaprilat, the active metabolite of quinapril, possesses the highest ACE binding affinity in both tissue and plasma.

- ◆ Tissue ACE and the endothelium appear to play important roles in the development of atherosclerosis. It is plausible that differences in ACE binding affinity could translate into differential clinical responses.

Inhibition of Vascular ACE:
Perindopril vs. Other ACE Inhibitors

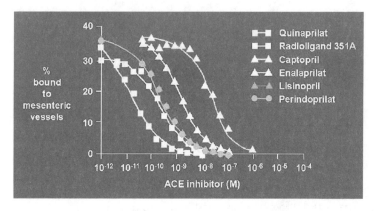

From Johnston Cl, et al. J Cardiovasc Pharmacol 1992;20(suppl B)S6-S11, with permission.

The RAAS is known to be a local endogenous tissue hormonal system with autocrine and paracrine effects. In the vessel wall, Ang II influences vasoconstriction and/or growth of SMCs, and it has been suggested that inhibition of ACE in vascular tissue may complement the beneficial systemic hemodynamic effects of ACE inhibition by producing favorable effects on vascular structure and function.

Shown here are curves representing the displacement of radiolabeled [125]I351A bound to vascular ACE in tissue from rat mesenteric vessels that have been exposed to different ACE inhibitors.

Inhibition of ACE by Perindopril in Endothelium and Adventitia of Human Internal Mammary Artery

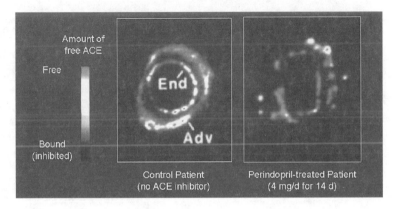

Adv = adventitia, End = endothelium.
From Zhuo, JL et al. Circulation. 1997;96:174-182, with permission

These autoradiographs from the Zhuo study, showing the internal mammary artery of a control patient compared with that of a perindopril-treated patient, illustrate perindopril's ACE-inhibiting effects.[59] The difference between the amount of free ACE in the control patient versus the perindopril-treated patient is immediately apparent, and the difference can be seen both at the level of the inner ring of endothelium and the outer ring of the adventitia.

Perindopril effectively penetrates the vascular wall to the depth of the adventitia, inhibiting ACE similarly in the endothelium and adventitia. Perindopril is effective in inhibiting ACE in vascular tissue.

ARBs and Endothelial Dysfunction: Treatment[6,27]

- ↑ BK

- ↑ NO

- Inhibit ET-1

- ↓ ROS/O_2^-

- ↓ EDCF

- Block TXA-A-II receptor

- Block deleterious effects of Ang-II

- ↑ Ang 1-7

- ↓ Homocysteine

- ↑ AC_1, ↑ C_1AC, ↑ C_2AC, ↓ PWV, ↓ AGI, ↓PP, ↑ AD, ↓ ASI

- ↓ MAU and proteinuria

- ↓ Uric acid (losartan)

- ↓ MLR

- Reduce atherosclerosis

Acute and Chronic Angiotensin-1 Receptor Antagonist Reverses Endothelial Dysfunction in Atherosclerosis

Abhiram Prasad, MB, MRCP; Theresa Tupas-Habib, BS;
William H. Schenke, BS; Rita Mincemoyer, RN;
Julio A. Panza, MD; Myron A. Waclawin, PhD,
Samer Ellaham, MD; Arshed A. Quyyumi, MD, FRCP

Circulation, 2000; 101:2349-2354

Effects of Angiotensin II, Before and After Losartan, on FVRI in Patients

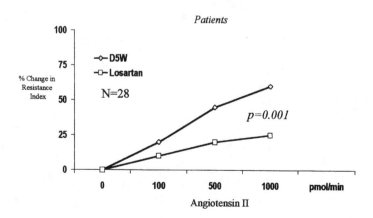

Prasad et al, Circulation 2000; 101:2349-2354

FVRI: Forearm Vascular Resistance Index

Effects of Angiotensin II, Before and After Losartan, on FVRI in Control Subjects

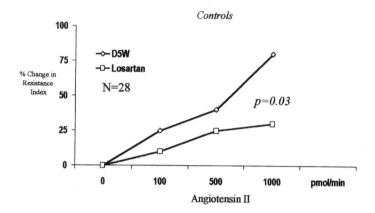

Controls

D5W
Losartan
N=28
p=0.03

% Change in Resistance Index

Angiotensin II

Effects of Sodium Nitroprusside, Before and After Losartan, in Patients

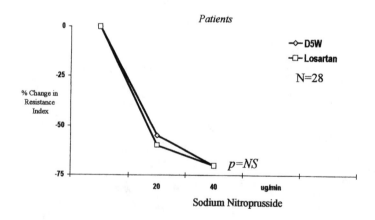

Patients

D5W
Losartan
N=28
p=NS

% Change in Resistance Index

Sodium Nitroprusside

Prasad et al, Circulation 2000; 101:2349-2354

FVRI: Forearm Vascular Resistance Index

Effects of Sodium Nitroprusside, Before and After Losartan, on FVRI in Control Subjects

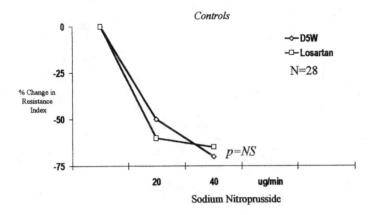

Effects of Acetylcholine, Before and After Losartan, on Percent Change in FVRI in Patients

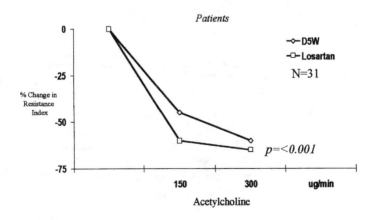

Prasad et al, Circulation 2000; 101:2349-2354

FVRI: Forearm Vascular Resistance Index

Effects of Acetylcholine, Before and After Losartan, on Percent Change in FVRI in Control Subjects

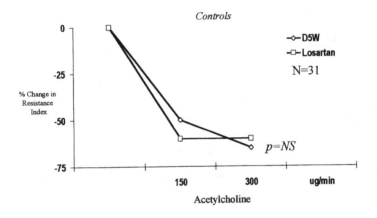

Effects of Losartan on Hyperemic Vasodilation Demonstrated as Change in FVRI in Patients

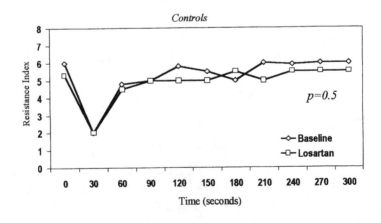

Prasad et al, Circulation 2000; 101:2349-2354

FVRI: Forearm Vascular Resistance Index

Effects of Losartan on Hyperemic Vasodilation Demonstrated as Change in FVRI in Control Subjects

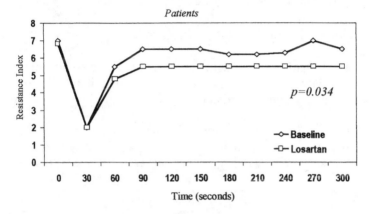

Prasad et al, Circulation 2000; 101:2349-2354

FVRI: Forearm Vascular Resistance Index

AT$_1$ Receptor Blockade and Endothelial Dysfunction

◆ Losartan therapy improved Ach-mediated microvascular dilation in atherosclerotic patients but not in control subjects.

◆ In contrast, responses to sodium nitroprusside were not altered, suggesting AT$_1$ receptor antagonism selectively improves endothelium-independent vasodilation in patients with atherosclerosis.

◆ The magnitude of improvement in Ach responses with parenteral Losartan correlated inversely with the initial response, suggesting improvement was greatest in those with the most depressed endothelial dysfunction.

Study Implications

In experimental atherosclerosis:

- ◆ AT_1 receptor blockade appears to have a protective effect.

- ◆ Mechanisms may include prevention of endothelial injury, augmentation of NO activity, inhibition of lipid peroxidation, and an antiproliferative effect.

- ◆ Observations that losartan improved endothelial function and NO activity suggest that AT_1 receptor antagonism ma also be antiatherogenic in patients with atherosclerosis.

Summary
Treatment of Hypertension
New Approach Based on Vascular Biology

Antihypertensive therapy must be directed at both reducing BP and improving ED and AC. Promoting vascular health by favorable effects on structure and function of the vasculature is associated with improved CV outcomes. The ARBs, ACEIs, and CCBs in comparative animal and human studies improve BP, ED, and AC better than diuretics and beta blockers.

Antilipid therapy with statins reduces stimulation of the AT_1R, increases eNOS, and NO, reduce oxLDL, reduces ROS and O^{2-}, improves EDV, and lowers BP slightly.

A combination of ARBs, ACEIs, CCBs, and statins in the hypertensive patient with hyperlipidemia is most likely to improve ED and AC, promote optimal vascular biologic effects, and reduce CV outcomes and target organ damage.

Chapter 17
Summary and Conclusions

1. Blood Vessel

The blood vessel should be the initial and primary target of both nonpharmacologic and pharmacologic therapy to prevent and treat atherosclerosis. Therapy should be aimed at the endothelium and the arterial wall.

2. Endothelial Dysfunction

ED is the initial and earliest event in vascular disease that eventually leads to functional and structural changes in the blood vessel. ED can occur in the absence atherosclerosis when only risk factors are present. ED precedes clinical atherosclerosis and events by many years.

ED occurs with loss of the balanced homeostatic mechanisms that determine vascular tone, growth thrombotic potential, inflammation, oxidation, and vessel wall permeability.

3. Endothelial Dysfunction (ED) and Arterial Compliance (AC)

Abnormalities or dysfunctions of the endothelium (ED) and the arterial wall (AC) are associated with increased future cardiovascular events. Correction and treatment of ED and abnormal AC reduce cardiovascular events.

4. Oxidative Stress

Oxidative stress is a major determinant of vascular damage, atherosclerosis and premature aging of the blood vessel.

5. Detection and Prevention of Vascular Disease

Noninvasive measurements of endothelial and vascular function (ED and arterial compliance) are necessary, important and will become standard clinical practice to detect vascular disease and institute appropriate lifestyle changes and pharmacologic therapy earlier, before the onset of clinical disease. In addition, prognostic information is obtained (i.e. CAPWA and EBT). CAPWA will complement the sphygmomanometer.

6. Holistic Approach to Blood Pressure

Understand and treat the mechanism, not the manifestation. Emphasis should be on pathophysiology of SBP, DBP, PP, CAPWA and arterial compliance. Relate the epidemiologic data to cardiovascular mechanics.

- ◆ Steady vs. pulsatile pressure as risk estimation.
- ◆ Different patterns of hypertension are due to different mechanisms.
- ◆ Pulse waveform is not uniform throughout the arterial tree.
- ◆ Central pressures are those that are physiologically relevant, and may or may not be the same as peripheral pressures.
- ◆ CAPWA and sphygmomanometer.

7. Hemodynamic Profiling

Hemodynamic profiling, using composite analysis of SBP, DBP and PP, is a superior risk predictor.

$$SBP = C_1 \text{ large conduit}$$
$$DBP = C_2 \text{ small arteries}$$
$$PP = \text{pulsatile flow}$$

8. New Definition of Hypertension

The blood pressure level at which there is NO NET increase in cardiovascular, cerebrovascular or renal morbidity or mortality.

9. Blood Pressure Goals Should be Reduced

An SBP of 110 mm Hg and a DBP of 70 mm Hg approach the plateau effect of neutral risk and TOD reduction in patients without concomitant risk factors. However, BP is a continuous variable and no specific cutoff points should be set in hypertensive or even normotensive patients.

10. Comprehensive Antihypertensive Therapy

Antihypertensive therapy must treat effectively more than BP

- ◆ Endothelial dysfunction
- ◆ Arterial compliance and vascular remodeling
- ◆ Non-traditional risk factors
- ◆ Emerging risk factors
- ◆ Traditional risk factors (DM, HLP)
- ◆ Risk markers (HSCRP, EBT)

11. Method of Blood Pressure Reduction

Method of blood pressure reduction determines endothelial vascular function and probably determines clinical outcomes of cardiovascular, cerebrovascular and renal TOD.

12. Vascular Structure and Function, BP and Outcome

Experimental studies in shr show some antihypertensive agents correct vascular structure with minor changes in BP but improved survival, suggesting the clinical outcomes may improve even in the absence of major BP reductions.[75]

13. Antihypertensive Drug Classes

The antihypertensive drug classes with the best overall profiles in vascular biology, blood pressure reduction, risk factor control, surrogate and clinical outcomes are:

> Calcium Channel Blockers (CCBs)
> Angiotensin Converting Enzyme Inhibitors (ACEIs)
> Angiotensin Receptor Blockers (ARBs)

14. Vascular Biology

Applied clinical application of the basic science as it related to vascular biology will be mandatory in order to select the best combination of therapy to improve endothelial function, arterial compliance and clinical outcome.

REFERENCES

1. Sherman DL. Exercise and endothelial function. Coron Artery Dis. 2000;11:117-122.
2. Hambrecht R, Wolf A, Gielen S, et al. Effect of exercise on coronary endothelial function in patients with coronary artery disease. N Engl J Med. 2000;342:454-460.
3. Caterina R. Endothelial dysfunctions: common denominators in vascular disease. Curr Opin Lipidol. 2000;11:9-23.
4. Contreras F, Rivera M, Vasquez, J, et al. Endothelial dysfunction in arterial hypertension. J Hum Hypertens. 2000;14 (suppl 1): S20-S25.
5. VanHoutie PM. How to assess endothelial function in human blood vessels. J Hypertens. 1999;17:1047-1058.
6. Ruschitzka F, Corti R, Noll G, Luscher TF. A rationale for treatment of endothelial dysfunction in hypertension. J Hypertens. 1999;17 (suppl):S25-S35.
7. Panza JA, Cardillo C. Potential mechanisms of endothelial dysfunction in patients with essential hypertension. J Hypertens. 1998;16 (suppl 8):S43-S48.
8. Intengan HD, Schiffrin EL. Role of endothelium in modulation of structural changes of small arteries in hypertension: effects of therapeutic intervention. J Hypertens. 1998:16 (suppl 8):S97-S101.
9. John S, Schmieder RE. Impaired endothelial function in arterial hypertension and hyperlipidemia: potential mechanisms and differences. J Hypertens. 2000;18:363-374.
10. Chun TH, Itoh H, Saito T, et al. Oxidative stress augments secretion of endothelium-derived relaxing peptides, C-type natriuretic peptide and adrenomedullin. J Hypertens. 2000;18:S75-S80.
11. Adams MR, Kinlay S, Blake J, et al. Atherogenic lipids and endothelial dysfunction: mechanisms in the genesis of ischemic syndromes. Annu Rev Med. 2000;51:149-167.
12. McIntyre M, Bohr DF, Dominiczak AF. Endothelial function in hypertension. The role of superoxide anion. Hypertension. 1999;34:539-545.
13. Pepine CJ. Clinical implications of endothelial dysfunction. Clin Cardiol. 1998;21:795-799.
14. Anderson TJ, Meredith IT, Charbonneau F. Endothelium-dependent coronary vasomotion relates to the susceptibility of LDL to oxidation in humans. Circulation. 1996;93:16471650.
15. Pedrinelli R, Dell'omo G, Bandinelli S, et al. Transvascular albumin leakage and forearm vasodilation to acetylcholine in essential hypertension. Am J Hypertens. 2000;13:256-261.
16. Klob S, Boulournie A, Mulsch A. Aging and chronic hypertension decrease expression of rat aortic soluble guanylyl cyclase. Hypertension. 2000;35:43-47.
17. Blankenship KA, Dawson CB, Aronoff GR, Dean WL. Tyrosine phosphorylation of human platelet plasma membrane CA^{2+}-atpase in hypertension. Hypertension. 2000;35:103-107.
18. Suuaidi JA, Hamasaki S, Higano ST, et al. Long-term followup of patients with mild coronary artery disease and endothelial dysfunction. Circulation. 2000,101:948-954.
19. Celermajer DS. How to measure endothelial functions in humans. Cardiol Rev. l999;DEC:1-7.
20. Yamakawa T, Tanaka S, Numaguchi K, et al. Involvement of rho-kinase in Angiotensin II induced hypertrophy of rat vascular smooth muscle cells. Hypertension. 2000;35[part 2]:313-318.
21. Hanke CJ, O'Brien T, Pitchard KA et al. Inhibition of adrenal cell aldosterone synthesis by endogenous nitric oxide release. Hypertension. 2000;35[part 2]:324-328.

220

22. Jackson WF. Ion channels and vascular tone. Hypertension. 2000;35[part 2]:173-178.

23. Smith IA, Lew RA, Shrimpton CN. A novel stable inhibitor of endopeptidases EC3.4.24.15 and 3.4.24.16 potentiates bradykinin-induced hypertension. Hypertension. 2000;35:626-630.

24. Parissis JT, Venetsanou, KF, Kalantzi MV. Serum profiles of Granulocyte- Macrophage colony stimulating factor and CC chemokines in hypertensive patients with or without significant hyperlipidemia. Am J Cardiol. 2000;85:777-779.

25. Pezza V, Bernardini F, Pezza E, et al. Study of supplemental oral L-arginine in hypertensives treated with enalapril plus hydrochlorothiazide. Am J Hypertens. 1998;Vol ll(No.10)Part 1:1267-1269.

26. Watanabe G, Tomiyama H, Doba N. Effects of oral administration of L-arginine on renal function in patients with heart failure. J Hypertens. 2000; 18:229-234.

27. Lind L, Granstam S, Millgard J. Endothelium-dependent vasodilation in hypertension: a review. Blood Pressure. 2000;9:4-15.

28. Goonasekera CDA, Shah V, Rees DD, Dillon MJ. Vascular endothelial cell activation associated with increased plasma asymmetric dimethyl arginine in children and young adults with hypertension: a basis for atheroma? Blood Press. 2000;9: 16-21.

29. Caterina RD, Liao JK, Libby P. Fatty acid modulation of endothelial activation. Am J Clin Nutr. 2000;71(suppl):213S-223S.

30. Cotton S, Vadala A, Mangano MT, et al. Endothelium derived factors in microalbuminuric and nonmicroalbuminuric essential hypertension. Am J Hypertens. 2000,13:172- 176.

31. Kobayashi N, Hara K, Watanade S, et al. Effect of imidapril on myocardial remodeling in L-name induced hypertensive rats is associated with gene expression of NOS and ACE mRNA. Am J Hypertension. 2000;13:199-207.

32. Hayashi S, Morishita R, Matsushita H. Cyclic AMP inhibited proliferation of human aortic vascular smooth muscle cells accompanied by induction of P53 and P21. Hypertension. 2000;35[part 2]:237-243.

33. Gros R, Chorazyczewski J, Meek M. G-protein-coupled receptor kinase activity in hypertension. Hypertension. 2000;35:38-42.

34. Dendorfer A, Wolfrum S, Schafer U, et al. Potentiation of the vascular response to kinins by inhibition of myocardial kininases. Hypertension. 2000;35:32-37.

35. Haller H, Kettritz R, Luft F. Endothelial cell markers in vasculitis. Kidney Blood Press Res. 1998;21:280-282.

36. Meerarani P, Ramadass P, Toborek M. Zinc protects against apoptosis of endothelial cells induced by linoleic acid and tumor necrosis factor. Am J Clin Nutr. 2000;71:81-87.

37. Riser BL, Cortes P, Lee J. Modelling the effects of vascular stress in mesangial cells. Curr Opin Nephrol Hypertens. 2000;9:43-47.

38. Petruzzelli L, Takami M, Humes D. Structure and function of cell adhesion molecules. Am J Med. 1999;106:467-476.

39. Etzioni A. Integrins: the molecular glue of life. Hosp. Pract. 2000;March 15:102-111.

40. Marul N, Offermann MK, Swerlicis R. Vascular cell adhesion molecule-1 (VCAM-1) gene transcription and expression are regulated through an antioxidant-sensitive mechanism in human vascular endothelial cells. J Clin Invest. 1993,92:1866-1874.

41. Price DT, Loscalzo J. Cellular adhesion molecules and atherogenesis. Am J Med. 1999;107:85-97.

42. Strong JP, Malcom GT, McMahan CA, et al. Prevalence and extent of atherosclerosis in adolescents and young adults. Implications for prevention from the pathobiological determinants of atherosclerosis in youth study. JAMA. 1999;281:727-735.

43. Enos WF, Holmes RH, Beyer T. Coronary disease among United States soldiers killed in action in Korea [landmark article]. JAMA. 1986;256:2859-2862.

44. Assman G, Cullen P, Schulte H. The Munster Heart Study (PROCAM). Eur Heart J. 1998;19(suppl A):A2-A11.

45. Holman RL, McGill HC, Strong JP, Geer JC. The natural history of atherosclerosis. Am J Pathol. 1958;34:209-235.

46. Stewart KG, Zhang Y, Davidge S. Aging increases PGHS-2-dependent vasoconstriction in rat mesenteric arteries. Hypertension. 2000;35:1242-1247.

47. Chester AH, Boriand JAA. Chymase-dependent angiotensin II formation in human blood vessels. J Hum Hypertens. 2000;14:373-376.

48. McCord JM. The evolution of free radicals and oxidative stress. Am J Med. 2000;108:652-659.

49. Dhalla NS, Temsah RM, Netticadan T. The role of oxidative stress in cardiovascular diseases. J Hypertens. 2000;18:655-673.

50. Wolf G. Free radical production and angiotensin. Curr Hypertens Reports. 2000;2:167-173.

51. Somers MT, Harrison DG. Reactive oxygen species and the control of vasomotor tone. Curr Hypertens Reports. 1999;1:102-108.

52. Usui M, Egashira K, Kitamoto S, et al. Pathogenic role of oxidative stress in vascular angiotensin converting enzyme activation in long-term blockade of nitric oxide synthesis in rats. Hypertension. 1999;34:546-551.

53. Laakso J, Mervaala E, Himberg JJ, et al. Increased kidney xantine oxidoreductase activity in salt-induced experimental hypertension. Hypertension. 1998;32:902906.

54. Romero JC, Reckelhoff JF Role of angiotensin and oxidative stress in essential hypertension. Hypertensin. 1999;34(part 2):943-949

55. Pedro-Botet J, Covas MI, Martin S, Rubies-Prat T. Decreased endogenous antioxidant enzymatic status in essential hypertension. J Hum Hypertens. 2000;14:343-345

56. Greene EL, Verlarde V, Jaffa AA. Role of reactive oxygen species in bradykinin-induced mitogen-activated protein kinase and C-FOS induction in vascular cells. Hypertension. 2000;35:942-947.

57. Ma GE, Mason DP, Young DB Inhibition of vascular smooth muscle cell migration by elevation of extracellular potassium concentration. Hypertension. 2000;35:948-951.

58. Lu G, Green L, Nagai T, Egan BM. Reactive oxygen species are critical in the oleic acid-mediated mitogenic signaling pathway in vascular smooth muscle cells. Hypertension. 1998;32:1003-1010.

59. Orie N, Zidek W, Tepel M. Reactive oxygen species in essential hypertension and non-insulin-dependent diabetes mellitus. Am J Hypertens. 1999;12:1169-1174.

60. Koska J, Syrova D, Blazicek P, et al. Malondialdehyde, lipofuscin and activity of antioxidant enzymes during physical exercise in patients with essential hypertension. J Hypertens. 1999;17:529-S35.

61. Mancini GBJ, Henry GC, Macaya C. Angiotensin-converting enzyme inhibition with quinapril improves endothelial vasomotor dysfunction in patients with coronary artery disease: the TREND (Trial on Reversing Endothelial Dysfunction) Study. Circulation. 1996;94:258-265.

62. Anderson TJ, Overhiser RW, Haber H, Charbonneau F, et al. A comparative study of four antihypertensive agents on endothelial function in patients with coronary disease [abstract]. J Am Coll Cardiol. 1998;31:327A.

63. Hornig B, Arakawa N, Haussman D, Drexler H. Differential effects on quinaprilat and enalaprilat on endothelial function of conduit arteries in patients with chronic heart failure. Circulation. 1998;98:2842-2848.

222

64. Oosterga M, Voors AA, Buikema H. Functional effects of ACE-inhibitors on angiotensin I conversion in human vasculature. J Am Coll Cardiol. 1998;31(suppl A):239A.

65. Fabre J-E, Rivard A, Magnin M, Isner JM. Angiotensin converting enzyme inhibition with quinaprilat stimulates angiogenesis in a rabbit model with hindlimb ischemia [abstract]. J Am Coll Cardiol. 1998;31(suppl A):239A.

66. Nissen SE, Gurley JC, Booth DC, DeMaria AN. Intravascular ultrasound of the coronary arteries: current applications and future directions. Am J Cardiol. 1992;69:18H-29H.

67. Pepine CJ. A symposium: endothelial function and cardiovascular disease: potential mechanisms and interventions. Am J Cardiol. 1998;82(10A):1S-64S.

68. Weir MR, Henrich WL. Theoretical basis and clinical evidence for differential effects of angiotensin-converting enzyme inhibitors and angiotensin II receptor subtype 1 blockers. Curr Opin in Nephrol and Hypertens. 2000;9:403-411.

69. Cohn JN. ACE-inhibition and vascular remodeling of resistance vessels. Vascular compliance and cardiovascular implications. Heart Disease. 2000;2:S2-S6.

70. Cohn JN. Vascular wall function as a risk marker for cardiovascular disease. J Hypertens. 1999;17(suppl S):S41-S44.

71. McVeigh GE, Bratteli CW, Morgan DT, et al. Age related abnormalities in arterial compliance identified by pressure pulse contour analysis. Aging and arterial compliance. Hypertension. 1999;33(6):1392-1398.

72. Vlachopoulos C, O'Rourke M. Diastolic pressure, systolic pressure or pulse pressure? Curr Hypertens Reports. 2000;2:271-279.

73. Glaser SP, Arnett DK, McVeigh GE, et al. Vascular compliance and cardiovascular disease. A risk or a marker? Am J Hypertens. 1997;10:1175-1189.

74. Glasser SP, Arnett DK, McVeigh GE, et al. The importance of arterial compliance in cardiovascular drug therapy. J Clin Pharmacol. 1998;38:202-212.

75. Park JB, Schiffrin EL. Effects of Antihypertensive therapy on hypertensive vascular disease. Curr Hypertens Reports. 2000;2:280-288.

76. Franklin SS. Is there a preferred antihypertensive therapy for isolated systolic hypertension and reduced arterial compliance? Current Hypertens Reps. 2000;2:253-259.

77. Buemi M, Corica F, Marino D, et al. Cardiovascular remodeling, apoptosis and drugs. Am J Hypertens. 2000;13:450-454.

78. Cohn J. Pathophysiologic and prognostic implications of measuring arterial compliance in hypertensive disease. Prog Cardiovasc Dis. 1999;41(6):441-450.

79. O'Rourke MF. Isolated systolic hypertension, pulse pressure and arterial stiffness as risk factors for cardiovascular disease. Curr Hypertens Rep. 1999;3:204-211.

80. Bulpitt CJ, Cameron JD, Rajkumar C. The effects of age on vascular compliance in man: which are the appropriate measures? J Hum Hypertens. 1999; 13:753-758.

81. Sharifi AM, Schiffrin EL. Apoptosis in vasculature of spontaneously hypertensive rats. Effect of an angiotensin converting enzyme inhibitor and a calcium channel antagonist. Am J Hypertens. 1998;11:1108-1116.

82. Bank AJ, Kaiser DR. Smooth muscle relaxation. Effects on arterial compliance, Distensibility, elastic module and pulse wave velocity. Hypertension. 1998;32:356-359.

83. Arnett DK, Boland LL, Evans GW, et al. Hypertension and arterial stiffness: the atherosclerosis risk in communities study. Am J Hypertens. 2000;13:317-323

84. Cockeroft JR, Webb DJ, Wilkinson IB. Arterial stiffness, hypertension and diabetes mellitus. J Hum Hypertens. 2000;14:377-380.

85. Franklin SS. Aging and hypertension: the assessment of blood pressure indices in predicting coronary heart disease. J Hypertens. 1999,17(suppl 5):S29-S36.

86. Baumbach GL, Chillon JM. Effects of angiotensin-converting enzyme inhibitors on cerebral vascular structure in chronic hypertension. J Hypertens. 2000;18(suppl):S7-S11.

87. Kuller LH, Sutton-Tyrrell K, Matthews KA. Blood pressure levels and measurement of Subclinical vascular disease. J Hypertens. 1999;17(suppl 5):S15-Sl9.

88. Malek AM, Alper SL, Izumo S. Hemodynamic shear stress and its role in atherosclerosis. JAMA. 1999;282(21):2035-2042.

89. Resnick N, Yahau H, Schubert S, et al. Signaling pathways in vascular endothelium activated by shear stress: relevance to atherosclerosis. Curr Opin in Lipidol. 2000;11:167177.

90. Kannel WB. Elevated blood pressure as a cardiovascular risk factor. Am J Cardiol. 2000;85:251-255.

91. Smulyan H, Safar ME. The diastolic blood pressure in systolic hypertension. Ann Intern Med. 2000;132;233-237.

92. Staessen JA, Gasowski J, Wang JG, et al. Risks of untreated and treated isolated systolic hypertension in the elderly: meta-analysis of outcome trials. Lancet. 2000;355:865-872.

93. Starmans-Kool, MJF, Kleinjans, HAJ, Lustermans, FAT, et al. Treatment of elderly patients with isolated systolic hypertension with isosorbide dinitrate in an asymmetric dosing schedule. J Hum Hypertens. 1998;12:557-561.

94. Black HR, Kuller LH, O'Rourke MF, et al. The first report of the systolic and pulse pressure (SYPP) working group. J Hypertens. 1999;17(suppl 5):S3-S14.

95. Blacher J, Staessen JA, Girerd X, et al. Pulse pressure not mean pressure determines cardiovascular risk in older hypertensive patients. Arch Intern Med. 2000;160:1085-1089.

96. Safar ME. Epidemiological aspects of pulse pressure and arterial stiffness. J Hypertens. 1999;17(suppl 5):S37-S40.

97. Busse R, Fleming I. Nitric oxide, nitric oxide synthase, and hypertensive vascular disease. Curr Hypertens Reports. 1999;1:85-88.

98. Stamler J. Nitric oxide in the cardiovascular system. Coron Artery Dis. 1999;10:273-276.

99. Soma M, Nakayama T, Kanmatsuse K. Nitric oxide synthase gene polymorphism and its influence on cardiovascular disease. Curr Opin Nephrol Hypertens. 1999;8:83-87.

100. Maxwell AJ, Cooke JP. The role of nitric oxide in atherosclerosis. Coron Artery Dis. 1999;10:277-286.

101. Zou AP, Cowley AW. Role of nitric oxide in the control of renal function an salt sensitivity. Curr Hypertens Reports. 1999;1:178-186.

102. Klahr S. The role of L-arginine in hypertension and nephrotoxicity. Opin Nephrol Hypertens. 1998;7:547-550.

103. Bhagat K, Vallance P. Effects of cytokines on nitric oxide pathways in human vasculature. Current Opinion in Nephrology and Hypertension. 1999;8:89-96.

104. Campbell DJ. Bioactive angiotensin peptides other than angiotensin II receptor antagonists. Epstein M, and Brunner HR (eds): Angiotension II Receptor Antagonists. Hanley and Belfus, Philadelphia, 2001.

105. Gimbrone MA, Topper JN. Biology of the vessel wall: endothelium. In Chien KR (ed): Molecular Basis of Cardiovascular Disease. Philadelphia, WB Saunders Company, 1999, pp 331-348.

106. Libby P, Hansson GK, Rober JS. Atherogenesis and inflammation. In Chien KR (ed): Molecular Basis of Cardiovascular Disease. Philadelphia, WB Saunders, 1999, pp 349-366.

107. Panza JA. Nitric oxide in hypertension. pp 158-165. In Oparil S, Weber MA (eds): Hypertension: A Companion to Brenner and Rector's: The Kidney. Philadelphia, WB Saunders, 2000, pp 158-165.

224

108. Oparil S, Weber MA. Hypertension: A Companion to Brenner and Rector's: The Kidney. Philadelphia, WB Saunders, 2000.
109. Fabiani ME, Dinh DT, Nassis L, Johnston CI. Angiotensin-converting enzyme: basic properties, distribution and functional role. In Weber MA (eds): Hypertension: A Companion to Brenner and Rector's: The Kidney. WB Saunders, 2000, pp 90-97.
110. Stary HC. Atlas of Atherosclerosis: Progression and Regression. New York and London, Parthenon, 1999.
111. Kannel WB, Blood pressure as a cardiovascular risk factor: prevention and treatment. JAMA. 1996;275:1572-1576.
112. Weber MA, Smith DHG, Neutel JM, Graettinger WF. Arterial properties of early hypertension. J Hum Hypertens. 1991;5:417-423.
113. Dzau VJ, Gibbons GH. Vascular remodeling: mechanisms and implications. J Cardiovasc Pharmacol. 1993;21(suppl 1):S1-S5.
114. Dzau, VJ. Tissue renin-angiotensin system in myocardial hypertrophy and failure. Arch Intern Med 1993;153:937-942.